AI in Healthcare

How Artificial Intelligence Is Changing
IT Operations and Infrastructure
Services

Rob Shimonski

WILEY

I dedicate this book to all the heroes whom I have had the honor to work with and support during the pandemic of 2020. You will always be remembered for your care, humanity, and unwavering support of communities in need. Thank you.

About the Author

Rob Shimonski is a technology executive specializing in healthcare IT for one of the largest health systems in America. In his role at Northwell Health, Rob is a decision maker and strategy planner for information systems operations and technology services. In his current role Rob is responsible for bringing operational support into the future with the help of new technologies such as cloud and artificial intelligence. His current focus is on AIOps. He's written dozens of books on many IT topics such as penetration testing, incident handling, cyberwarfare, and the deployment of advanced network and security tools and technologies.

With the onset of "too much" data to handle, it's obvious that something needs to be done to bridge the gap between healthcare operations and leveraging the data to improve patient experience and clinical support. With AI and operations (AIOps), this can be done through the connection of real-time event correlation and automation of responses to help restore critical IT functions. Other benefits can be found in customer (patient, clinician) experience outcomes. Rob works to lead this transformation from the forefront of bridging the business with the technology assets needed to create a technical health road map of new opportunities.

Rob works to connect business goals, build on customer/patient/clinician experience, and help strategize (and deploy) operational delivery systems to create a cycle of continuous improvement, with the potential to invent new markets within pre-existing healthcare technology architecture.

Rob's experience has been extremely diverse but always focused on innovation and developing new solutions to create efficiency and bringing forth better outcomes through the use of technology solutions. Rob can be found online at www.shimonski.com.

About the Technical Editor

Ted Coombs is a polymath futurist, technologist, and author of 24 technology books. His career in tech started in the 1970s as a laser engineer and roboticist. He began working in AI in 1983 for the Cleveland Clinic. He is one of the founders of modern computer forensics and today is also known for his knowledge of AIOps and DataOps. He is also an accomplished musician and fine artist.

Acknowledgments

I would like to personally thank all of my colleagues, leaders, and teams at Northwell Health. The teams I lead and am a part of are some of the best in the industry, and without them, we would never be able to accept and complete the challenges we confront day by day. From deploying new technologies to supporting the operation to bringing innovation to the forefront—it truly is one big team that makes it all happen. Although the list could be infinite, I would like to thank the leaders I report to for their amazing guidance. Most importantly, Michael J. Dowling, chief executive officer of Northwell Health, for his leadership not only during the pandemic but for all the time I have worked for Northwell Health. His ability to be innovative and tackle operational issues head on and lead from the front is what is most inspiring of any leader, especially of a CEO. I would also like to thank my leaders—CIO John Bosco, CTO Dr. Purna Prasad, AVPs Mike Tralli, Pat Clark, and Vince Pawlowski, and my managers Bob Setti, Gail McGarry, Eric Lindner, and Peter Cheung—for being amazing at what they do every day. This list is not exhaustive, but for the sake of brevity, I would like to offer an extended thank-you to the many great people I have worked with and have had the honor to lead in this organization. I can't thank all of you enough.

I would also like to extend my thanks to the amazing team at Wiley. First and foremost, Kenyon Brown for listening to my request to make this book and sharing in my excitement. I remember our first phone call about it and how we both would express how awesome it would be to make this book, and now here it is! Thanks for allowing me to do this. I would like to extend a debt of gratitude to my project editor Kelly Talbot, who basically helped me create this book every step of the way. Your help, insight, and assistance are very much appreciated, and I can't thank you enough for your efforts on making this book a great book. I would also like to thank Ted Coombs, my technical editor, for helping to point out a few things that would make this book even better: thank you! I would like to round out the publishing acknowledgments with a big thank-you for my literary agent, Carole Jelen, vice president of Waterside Productions. I feel like we have been working together for so many years that you know not only how to point out good ideas but how to market them and myself like a pro. Thank you.

Lastly, I would like to thank my family for their support while writing this book. I like to believe that I am present in their lives at all times, but when it comes to work and then doing a book project in the evenings and weekends, sometimes that takes some extra time away from "fun," so thank you. Thanks to my parents, Bob and Barbara; my son, Dylan; my daughter, Vienna; and especially my wife, Allison, who always believed in me, believes in me, believes in what I do, and most importantly believes in what I am going to do next. I love you.

—Rob Shimonski

Contents at a Glance

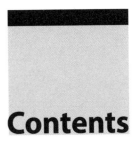

Contents

Introduction

Today's systems, network, data, and critical infrastructure are all dependent on becoming more efficient and "self-aware," while also self-healing. Artificial intelligence (AI) in operational models has become the de facto standard of how services will be designed and deployed in the future. This fusion of AI and operations has spawned the newly infamous acronym AIOps. As operations becomes the foundation of integrity that critical enterprise systems rely on, it's no mystery that AIOps has become incredibly popular as of late.

Service delivery is the lifeblood of all companies looking to be and remain competitive. This is especially true in highly critical services such as those delivered by healthcare where lost time, mistakes, and red tape impact the patient experience negatively. With more push toward zero downtime and less impact to 24/7/365 systems, having the intelligence to weather this storm is one of the most exciting prospects turned reality of our time and can be fully realized with the use of AI-based systems. Using this book, you will not only learn about AI and its importance, but be given practical examples and advice on how to actually deploy it in your environment to achieve these positive outcomes. It is also within this book that years of experience not only in other verticals but in the specific nature of healthcare delivery becomes evident as you progress through the chapters.

In this publication we explore what AI and ML are and how they are used in companies today. While this book covers machine learning and artificial intelligence concepts in depth, it also covers the practicality of deploying them into your enterprise. Another critical concept that remains a constant through this book is what AI and ML concepts are and how they apply to the myriad of tools, systems, and services offered today where corporate executives and technical engineers need to understand the "how to" when they need to make a decision and deploy the correct toolsets for the best outcomes. There is too much confusion and not enough real data surrounding how to select a good tool (or tools) to get this accomplished in operational departments today. This book also focuses on the primary sector where AI and ML are creating some of the biggest impacts today: healthcare IT (HIT).

Some of the key target areas that this book covers in detail include the foundations of AI and ML and what you need to know to be able to recommend and then deploy the technology. Concepts such as AI and how it fused with IT operations and specifically healthcare IT are covered in depth. There is also a deep look into clinical operations and how infrastructure services and IT operations support the clinical role and how both can interact successfully for mutual advantage, leverage AI for maximum potential, and increase successful outcomes for clinicians and their client or patients. Key target areas include but are not limited to the following:

- Healthcare IT
- AI clinical operations
- AI operational infrastructure
- Project planning
- Metrics, reporting, and service performance
- AIOps in automation
- AIOps cloud operations

The goal of this book is to help build confidence in deploying a technology that will radically change how operations are done today. It requires understanding the versions of available AIOps platforms and systems, the vendors involved, and what infrastructure is needed. Once it is completely defined and understood from this perspective, we will explore applications of AI and ML in specific settings (or verticals) such as healthcare and how to strategize for these deployments in a cost-effective manner. The key to doing this well is to know how to use project management fundamentals to create a successful project. Project planning is the primary focus here with all of the planning done up front before the rollout to maximize the ROI for these large-scale deployments of technology. In the healthcare setting, there is an enterprise operational use of AI, and there is a clinical use, and it's important to know how they differ and how they can be integrated. This is where true innovation takes place. Although the book does cover many concepts of clinical AI and how it works in the grand scheme of IT, operational use of AI for the integrity of IT and healthcare assets, proactive and automated systems based on learned data, how to gauge service performance, and ultimately how to better deliver services (service delivery) of healthcare via IT is the primary focus and how it relates to AIOps.

Lastly, the book will cover a brief history of AI from 30 years ago until today, including where it came from, where it grew from, and ultimately where it is going (the direction it is heading). It is important to know how AI, ML, and AIOps work with cloud technologies, IoT, and other emerging technologies so that there are no missed opportunities due to lack of knowledge. It is the goal of this book to prepare you not only to understand but to be successful at a current and future rollout, implementation, and ongoing support framework for operations using AIOps in your healthcare setting.

What Does This Book Cover?

This book covers the following topics:

Chapter 1, "Healthcare IT and the Growing Need for AI Operations," opens the book by providing a brief but thorough history on artificial intelligence (AI), machine learning (ML), and healthcare information technology (HIT). The chapter brings focus to current operations and how HIT is expanding and growing and how the digital transformation of providing healthcare requires a more focused view on technology operations, infrastructure services, providing care through technology, and how to innovatively change the digital footprint to provide reliable services for patient care. Other important topics covered are how artificial intelligence operations (AIOps) brings these different functions together and gives the users of the technology more insight into their technology investments.

Chapter 2, "AI Healthcare Operations (Clinical)," builds on what was covered in Chapter 1 by providing a different view into AI and ML and how it directly impacts clinical operations. Topics such as intelligent cloud, data analytics, informatics, convergence, and other methods to merge innovative efforts between technology support and clinical operations under the AIOps umbrella are discussed in great detail. Other topics include the need for security in the clinical technology space and why service performance is critical to providing reliable patient care on stable systems.

Chapter 3, "AI Healthcare Operations (Operational Infrastructure)," covers the strategy pillars and fundamentals required to get started with developing, strategizing, conceptualizing, and selecting products and vendors for your AIOps deployment in your organization. Topics covered include creating the project scope for vendor selection; selecting platforms, products, and services from tool vendors; and sizing the request correctly. Product vendors such as ServiceNow, Dynatrace, and Splunk are covered to help you design the correct deployment for your enterprise. Other topics include event and fault management and how these functions tie into advanced workflow and automation topics to help bridge the gap between AI and manual intervention.

Chapter 4, "Project Planning for AIOps," builds on the concepts learned in Chapter 3 when project scope was introduced to help with vendor selection. In this chapter, you learn how to finish building the project plan and how to bring AIOps into enterprises consisting of large infrastructures. Project management concepts are covered, such as how to select a good project manager, how to build the project team (and why it's critical to success), what a good project plan looks like, and how to build a program into your portfolio. The chapter also discusses deploying AIOps in your environment using a project plan, communicating status updates, and keeping executives informed of project milestones.

Chapter 5, "Using AI for Metrics, Performance, and Reporting," details what you need to know post-deployment. Once you have deployed AIOps and are running it in your organization, you need to ensure your return on investment (ROI) by covering service performance metrics, KPIs, CSFs, and other important metrics that show how your investment in AIOps is creating a positive impact in both your IT environment and your clinical environment. Using AI for metrics, performance, and reporting allows you to feel confident in your AIOps platform by looking at how well it is performing and by building and viewing dashboards that help tell a story of success. Other tools helpful to building and showing metrics are covered as well as what you can pull directly from tools such as ServiceNow and Splunk.

Chapter 6, "AIOps and Automation in Healthcare Operations," discusses how to develop advanced automation for real-world healthcare operations. By looking at tools such as ServiceNow and others, building processes, designing workflows, and other automation functions, you get a full understanding of how this helps to reduce outages, increase visibility, and increase the availability of systems. Through warning detection, incident engagement, and event handling, the framework for automation is covered in great detail to help create good-quality control in your environment. The chapter includes advanced discussions on how to create and build machine learning into process automation, how artificial intelligence self-learns, and other advanced service intelligence topics.

Chapter 7, "Cloud Operations and AIOps," covers the movement of operations from in-house solutions to hosted solutions with product vendors or other managed service providers. Regardless of where you decide to host your platform, the details of doing so are covered in depth. Other topics that are covered are the strategy of moving an operation into the cloud from an in-house solution, what offerings and service types are available, how to do a request for proposal (RFP), when cloud should (and shouldn't be) an option, how to manage your instance in the cloud, and what you need to know about security of the cloud within a healthcare environment.

Chapter 8, "The Future of Healthcare AI," brings about the next offerings in AI and ML technology to include telehealth services, the Internet of Things (IoT), and the continual merge of clinical operations and the reliance on IT systems. Other topics include Big Data, DataOps, analytics, and informatics, which are crucial in today's health environments where the size of stored (and protected) data is growing exponentially every day. The use of AI, ML, and AIOps to manage this data and these new technologies is becoming more and more important, and vendors are looking at new ways to build their services that allow for these innovative drivers to develop into AI solutions for enterprise management and monitoring.

Chapter 9, "The Convergence of Healthcare AI Technology," covers more advanced topics that include convergence of critical systems managed by AIOps. As more and more healthcare operations rely on IT systems, the deployment of overarching enterprise management and monitoring solutions becomes more and more apparent as well as important. In this chapter, we cover AIOps for systems integration and overall systems management; the convergence of AI, HIT, and HIE; and other systems such as IoT end points.

Lastly, the appendix, "Sample AIOps Use Cases and Examples," shows real-world examples of problems in the healthcare environment in the form of use cases that are solved by many of the topics in this book. Understanding what this book covers can help provide guidance on how to navigate real challenges such as outages that can be healed by AI technologies to reduce impact to the system and potentially save lives in the process of doing so.

Reader Support for This Book

If you believe you've found a mistake in this book, please bring it to our attention. At John Wiley & Sons, we understand how important it is to provide our customers with accurate content, but even with our best efforts an error may occur.

To submit your possible errata, please email it to our Customer Service Team at wileysupport@wiley.com with the subject line "Possible Book Errata Submission."

Healthcare IT and the Growing Need for AI Operations

Shall we play a game?
—Joshua (from *WarGames*)

In today's ever-changing business model of do it faster, do it better, and do it without flaws, there needs to be a balance between those who create the technology and technology having a mind of its own. As in the famous quote "Shall we play a game?" healthcare operations is anything but a game and lives hang in the balance. In today's organizations, that balance is being established as technologies such as artificial intelligence (AI) are being implemented. There needs to be a way to do more work efficiently and with greater intelligence while still ensuring that the work is performed correctly. With the boom of healthcare advancements and the need to keep up with technological change, those who rely on all of the newest technology for clinical operations need an enterprise system that ensures that the technology continues to work for us and not against us. That combination of technology and clinical advancement comes in the form of a successful merging of intelligence and strategy, using the correct tools for the job, and planning and designing a platform that works for you, not against you. This is AI operations (AIOps) in healthcare.

This chapter explores the healthcare market and how technology continually changes it, specifically within the realm of AIOps. In these pages I will discuss the growing need for technology in this space, how healthcare has been fundamentally (and forever) changed by the digital landscape, and all of the specifics revolving around AIOps. This includes how AIOps is being used to create efficiency, reduce downtime, increase time to respond to issues, improve the ability to automate efforts to reduce waste and time spent doing computation work, and ultimately create better customer experiences for all patients, clinicians, and everyone involved in the healthcare space.

In the first portion of this chapter, I will cover the basic history of artificial intelligence (AI) and machine learning (ML). Although some could say we have always been in a perpetual state of "machine learning" for as long as we have had machines and in a constant state of computational (or artificial) intelligence as long as we could compute things, there are some significant milestones in the ML and AI timeline. For one, as long as we have been playing games, there has always been a study of game theory and outcomes through games. Many military and war strategists believed in game theory, and this became even more apparent when IBM began testing ML theory with gaming to produce the first machine learning game in the 1950s when someone played checkers and the program was able to learn from the outcomes of the game, the players' choices, and so on. I think this real story was likely the predecessor to the movie *WarGames* decades later. Checkers, chess, backgammon, and other games were all tested to see how a machine could learn.

As more and more technology (machines) was created and advanced, the same questions and theories were applied to it. When cars were made, how could we get them to learn? What about if we made a robot? Could it learn? The same theories from a long time ago all waited until technology caught up and provided for computers, robotics, and other major technological advancements that could be fused with machines to allow them to learn. Once computers were added to cars, then cars could start to learn. Now we drive in cars that can predict a possible crash and take action. This development went way beyond the abilities of game theory, but it should be noted that the mathematical equations, usage, and logic behind it still remained the same. It was only advancing as quickly as the technology did and was expanded on.

Another major installment of ML and AI development came with the World Wide Web (WWW), the Internet, and the Internet of Things (IoT), where the interconnected nature and development of all of technology was able to fuse and share data as well as save it. The saving of large quantities of data (or big data theory) allowed for more math to be applied for machine learning capabilities. Also, the growth of large-scale search engines (like Google) continued to allow for even more ML and AI abilities due to the analytics that could be applied to "customize" an experience for every user. Augmented reality (AR), wearable technology, DNA collection, mobile technologies, social media, and so many other advancements bring us to a stage in life where ML and AI are able to be used not only in any one of these advancement areas but also across them as they too interconnect.

This is where we begin our journey into the development and fundamental layout of AI, ML, and AIOps in the healthcare world. Healthcare is the largest user of all the technologies I just mentioned and the biggest connector of intelligence usage to increase the use of treatment, medicine, and patient satisfaction. We now need to know how to keep all of these systems running and available, continue to perform their computations, and allow for the continued interconnection and learning to provide the best care possible now and in the future.

A Brief History of AI and Healthcare

No industry is bigger, more important, more dynamic, and exploding with change than healthcare. Some may argue that it is similar to the industrial revolution in its transformative scope. The electronic medical record (EMR) and other technological advancements are changing the way we see, deliver, and expect to receive our healthcare. One of the most interesting things about the healthcare industry is we are all our own clients, customers, and patients, which makes our industry unique in that it is something we hope we never have to use but absolutely must have in the form of benefits to cover our families and ourselves. Working in this field can be the most rewarding experience one can have, and seeing its growth and being a part of its transformation can be a once-in-a-lifetime experience.

As the healthcare field grows in every aspect, we must consider the technology used to bolster this revolutionary expansion. We call this technological field *healthcare information technology* (also known as healthcare IT or HIT). In this chapter, I will explain healthcare IT, some of its history, and why technology has expanded it exponentially. I will also start to talk about the need for another popular and growing technological advancement called *artificial intelligence* (AI). Beyond that, we will bridge the two technologies—healthcare IT and AI—and explore a third topic called *healthcare operations* so we can create a fusion between them all, which is known today as *artificial intelligence operations* (AIOps). Let's begin our journey in this chapter and this book by starting from the beginning, which is the expansion of healthcare as we know it today.

THE CORONAVIRUS AND COVID-19

When the coronavirus (COVID-19) pandemic spread around the world in 2020, it affected the world of medicine in a dramatic way. As I will cover in Chapter 8, "The Future of Healthcare AI," there have been radical changes to the use, delivery, and expectations of healthcare service.

With guidance by the World Health Organization (WHO), Centers for Disease Control and Prevention (CDC), and local, state, and government leaders, the world population had to make radical changes to slow the spread of COVID-19. For one, all healthcare systems (hospitals, practices, etc.) needed to find ways to reconfigure to handle the surge into the emergency department (ED) and intensive care unit (ICU) areas of the system. Temporary facilities were set up, and many new ways of practicing emergency medicine were considered. New medications, new treatments, and a world of new research into finding a cure were put in place. The world actively worked to slow the spread and focus on a cure. New technologies emerged, the importance of keeping systems up and running found a renewed priority level, and the use of older technologies saw a resurgence, like telemedicine.

Healthcare IT Expansion and Growth

The radical expansion and growth of IT and healthcare IT was just the beginning. It provided the needed building blocks to get to where we are today so that we can collect data in large amounts (*big data*), analyze it, and make predictions and assessments to create better outcomes. Big data analysis helps our knowledge and handling of population health, the need to reduce hospital stays, what can be done inside an acute versus nonacute facility, and how to make predictions on outcomes in a geographic area. An example of a prediction in an area would be how seasonal flu may impact certain areas and why that may be. This only scratches the surface of what we can leverage big data for.

To get to this point, we needed to get all data into the computer systems. By creating the electronic medical record (EMR) and having clinical staff adding this data to these systems, the building block was in place to start expanding this practice across all health systems. This provided many benefits, one of which was leveraging the resources of the many instead of the few. The increasing cost of healthcare put a lot of stress on smaller hospitals that could no longer afford to continue to build technical systems while still expanding their operations outside of information technology. Other important factors include (but are not limited to) security, risk, and compliance where privacy became paramount by law.

Compliance, meaningful use, regulatory bodies, inspections, laws and even the dominance of the Health Insurance Portability and

Accountability Act (HIPAA) passed by Congress in 1996 continued to drive more and more healthcare providers to join forces with others to share resources so they could stay afloat. One of the many benefits was the ability to leverage the administrative functions (like technology) between providers, clinicians, healthcare facilities, practices, hospitals, and even insurance. Another advantage was the chance to scale up on all of these shared resources, which allowed hospitals and practices to share operational data so that they could model best practices and standards to keep all of these technology systems operational, resilient, and well-positioned for future innovation.

BIG DATA AND ITS IMPORTANCE

Data is the fundamental building block to everything that we do in technology. Think of a simple, traditional network. A network is useless unless you have something to share. Would you spend all of this money to set up countless connections simply for the sake of having connections? Of course not. You need to share data from printers, faxes, email, text messages, and files.

Big data is the same building block for AI, ML, and AIOps. Without data, what are you collecting, and why would you need it in the first place? The key to doing mathematical and computational analysis is to find ways to solve equations, and when you apply large volumes of data and a plan for finding trends, you wind up with predictive analytics. Analytics is what you do to mine the data for whatever specific information you need. So, if you are trying to see where there are systematic flu outbreaks in an area and why the flu outbreaks are occurring there, you need to collect data, analyze it, and create a mathematical prediction based on the trends. Big data is the large-scale collection of data that would need to be mined to identify trends when you conduct your analysis.

Data Overload

The many sources of data and the need for it to be shared started to become overwhelming. IT environments continued to grow exponentially, outpacing the underlying resources needed to run them. For example, extremely large enterprise storage system platforms with terabytes of space and high-speed delivery became essential to keep up with the needs for storing and leveraging data, particularly for the data scientists who looked at, analyzed, and computed this data (big data) for many use cases.

Data overload is a potential issue. You can collect a ton of data and not know what to do with it because you lack the strategy, tools, understanding, applications, services, or staffing needed to unlock what is within it. You may also run into issues where you cannot collect, store, mine, or access in a reliable way the large data sets you collect. You may also run into issues with sharing these large data sets. For example, I have seen in the past where research teams conducting important studies could not share files with other research teams remotely because of their large size. What people may not know is that (as an example) a magnetic resonance imaging (MRI) file with large slicing capability could be terabytes in size depending on the resolution of the file in use. When sharing hundreds of these over a typical 10 megabit connection with virtual private network (VPN) encryption, you could expect issues!

Unorganized data is another potential issue. When you work with data, you need to tag it correctly so that it can be accessed via field searches in databases. If you do not tag it correctly, when you run scans to find keywords or other criteria, you may not find what you are looking for, or worse, you may miss large portions of data, which can skew or create kurtosis of your results.

Unusable data is a related concern, meaning the data is missing entirely (orphaned), misunderstood (outliers), or corrupted and therefore unusable.

In any of these cases, you can have a data grooming exercise conducted to make sure that a sample set of the data shows that these problems may or may not exist and be fixed if possible. This is generally part of an organization's master data management (MDM) program. Regardless of what state your data is in, you need to recognize that it could be problematic and cause issues in your deployments, use of AI and ML, and other future endeavors of innovation. One of the most important things to consider when conducting any mathematical or computational exercise is that your data is usable and trustworthy.

CLEANING UP YOUR DATA WITH MDM

Data is the fundamental building block to everything that we do in technology. The best way to handle your data is to start fresh and make sure that your organization utilizes a master data management (MDM) program. An MDM is more of a governance committee made up of both technology and business leaders that puts rules into effect on how all company data will be tagged, listed, used, controlled, stored, and named (conventions). This includes identifying who has access, who owns what data, who maintains the data, and who ensures the lifelong accuracy and accountability of all data shared within the company. Without a program of this kind, you will run into issues later when your data grows so huge that it will take large project-like efforts and create massive disruption to address these and other issues. If you plan on working with data (which is the building block of AI and ML and thus AIOps), make sure that you know what the state of your data is before you begin innovative projects that require the use of big data.

Digital Transformation of Healthcare

The digital transformation of healthcare takes two paths: the clinical and the operational. Although I will cover them both in this chapter, the focus of the book really only goes deeply into one of these two paths. Although they are intertwined, they are in fact different when it comes to their stated purpose and scope. Make no mistake, they are both connected, and one may argue that you can't have one without the other. Case in point, if you do not have a stable environment in which to work (AIOps), how can you have a platform to conduct informatics to prevent illness or disease? On the contrary, why would you have a large AIOps platform if you weren't doing this type of the work in the first place? You can also argue that without the development and growth of AI and ML over the years, the fusion of this technology into newer tools like event and fault management platforms, service management tools, and help desk systems would be pointless when it comes to building on AI and its benefits. As you can see, they are both interdependent.

To further explain these two paths, path 1 is the clinical informatics space where AI and ML are used to do informatics work. Big data and its dissection are the future of clinical healthcare. As we collect more and more data, successfully analyzing it allows us to predict behaviors, solve clinical problems, create cures, or create new treatment plans. Looking at this data can tell you historically how many times the flu came through an area and at what impact rate so you can make sure that you market the flu shot effectively or logistically ensure that you have sufficient vaccines in that area. The use of this data is important to innovation and research for moving healthcare forward into the future.

NOTE   For the clinical side of AI, ML, informatics, and using data to create positive outcomes, there is a natural fear that the storage and usage of this data would somehow create a privacy concern. However, all healthcare systems, providers, and users of this data are mandated to only use copies of the data that have been de-identified for use. This means all identifying data that can link any medical data to a patient by name or any other form of ID is removed completely before any data is used to study. This allows for privacy to remain intact.

Path 2 is the AIOps path where AI and ML are the focus of using enterprise platform systems that keep all of the data up and running alongside the EMR and every other clinical system, application, program, and system in use in the health provider environment.

For example, consider a patient needing to go in for an annual checkup, complete with routine blood work and urine sample. The doctor reviews the results of blood and urine tests to give the patient an assessment of the current state of their health. The doctor may also look at the patient's chart to see what they are predisposed to, their family history, their age, and many other factors before giving advice, a clinical path to follow, medications, or a referral to a specialist for further work. The patient's chart is reviewed to see what their last checkup or blood labs showed, and trends and patterns are examined so that nothing is missed. Various systems support the bloodwork lab, the urinalysis lab, the pharmacies, the specialists, the patient's historic files, the patient's current general condition, the ability to recognize patterns and predispositions, and the ability to project potential areas of concern, and AI and ML play a role in synchronizing and coordinating all of this data.

One of the reasons why understanding this is so important is that it sets the basis for keeping all of these operations up, running, stable, and operational. All of this technology must be highly available, recoverable from outage or disaster, and manageable. This can be done through traditional methods, but it can also be done with artificial intelligence. There are pros and cons to both, and we will explore these considerations throughout the book. Remember, the reason we want to design and set up an enterprise system like AIOps is so you, your family, your community, and your world can get the quality healthcare you expect and, in some cases, demand. If any of these systems are down, not operational, or corrupted, you can get delayed care, no care, or, in some rare cases, the wrong care, which can bring about life-altering experiences.

WARNING When dealing with a pandemic like COVID-19, the stability of infrastructure, the integrity of systems, and the reliability of key applications are beyond mission critical. They are always a priority, but with the need to keep healthcare workers focused on providing clinical care during such a dire crisis, the use of AIOps can be instrumental if deployed correctly. You need to strategize, configure, plan, deploy, and use AIOps to achieve that goal.

The Science of Healthcare Innovation

So, with all of this technology, what are we really striving to do? Much like Maslow's hierarchy of needs, we want to reach enlightenment and integrity. Once we have learned how to survive and take care of the fundamentals such as stability and integrity, we ultimately want to innovate. Innovation is the hallmark of any civilization that has moved to the highest stages of self-enlightenment.

With healthcare, the goal will be to have healthcare IT systems that run 24/7/365 with a five nines (99.999%) uptime and immediate resilience to any disaster whether technological, weather-based, military, or biological. We also want to reduce cost, waste, our environmental footprint, and our need to react to system issues. Lastly, we want to create efficiency, innovation, and the ability to rely on the systems we deploy and use. That's a lot to ask for, right? Well, this is the underlying goal that has spurred the entire market called AIOps. AIOps provides the ability to do everything I just said and more. With AIOps, your key systems will remain stable, and intelligent decisions will be made through machine learning to reduce impact related to downtime. Downtime impacts your ability to innovate.

To have innovation, we need our experts focused on their jobs. They should not be waiting for systems to recover from outages. They should not be working on how to connect users to systems as they recover. Our clinical experts shouldn't be using pen and paper during an outage and then afterward painstakingly entering that information to the EMR without a single data error. All of this is a waste of time and energy that creates missed opportunities for greatness. It also increases the potential for error.

Can we remove all of this waste and create innovation that we can all benefit from? The emergence of a technology platform that delivers AIOps promises to fulfill this role, among other things. Does it come with its own issues? Yes, and I will break them down and how to overcome them throughout this book. Regardless, the biggest goal of AIOps today is to create the ability to not have to manage failing systems and give that time back to those who would use it to create magic like innovative new healthcare solutions.

NOTE   There are many roles an IT expert can play in healthcare IT such as analyst, data scientist, technical professional, systems engineer, risk manager, and so on. Everyone in IT should be enjoined in AIOps, and all parties should be stakeholders to any project where AIOps is deployed and used in an enterprise. Others who are to be involved would be any clinicians, providers, or other staff who will use the systems. Including their voices helps ensure that systems will be developed and implemented reliably in your enterprise.

Artificial Intelligence in Healthcare

Before we can really delve into the platforms that deliver AIOps, other supporting platforms, offerings, designs, strategies, and use cases, you should have a firm understanding of the fundamental concepts of artificial intelligence, machine learning, operations research (OR), and other technologies that I will refer to throughout this book.

First, artificial intelligence is exactly how it sounds. You have a computer system (or form of technology) that is able to learn, grow smarter, or be self-aware. It has "intelligence" between its programming language and expected behavior. This is a far cry from the Cyberdyne Systems' Skynet in the *Terminator* movies. Will we one day have the type of adaptable, self-aware, artificial intelligence technology system like we see in science fiction? We don't know. However, for here and now, the answer is no, we have nothing like that. Today's AI is not Skynet. AI today is still in its infancy, and while it is mature in the sense that we have adapted it into many of our technology systems, the term *artificial intelligence* is more of a play on words than a truly conscious technology system.

In simple terms, current AI can be thought of as computer technology such as programming languages, applications, and systems that emphasize fabricated, simulated intelligence through patterns and trends. It is not conscious, but it is programmed to be intelligent. I think this is an important distinction to make right up front to make sure that you are working from the beginning with the correct definition and expectations.

As we develop AI systems, we can think of them as behaving as if they have consciousness. In doing so, it can help to further divide AI into hard AI and soft AI (also known as strong AI and weak AI). Soft AI is simple. It is usually purpose-built and performs a single or simple function. This can be thought of as a program that you operate such as a game that tracks and learns your skills, patterns, and game-playing behaviors. Hard AI is something more complex with deeper programming, abilities, functions, and architecture. A great example of hard AI would be Google Brain. Google Brain is a hard-AI, deep-learning, AI-based research program formed in the early 2010s by Google that incorporates the concepts of machine learning with the large-scale computing resources of an enterprise as large as Google. Hard AI such as this can be more successful at simulating intelligence because of the complexity and power scaled behind it.

Either way, whether hard or soft, AI is still something that needs to be developed, worked on, built, deployed, and managed, and once everything starts to really work well, it needs to be managed some more. This is an important point to keep in mind as you embark on your journey into the world of AI in healthcare. AI requires real time and effort. So, now that we have covered AI, how does machine learning fit in?

Machine learning is the science behind the AI machine. ML can be thought of as the mathematical algorithms, statistics, underlying models, and data that powers AI. ML can be seen as a subset or component of AI where AI is what is used to make decisions and ML is what gives AI the ability to learn new things to make decisions about. ML has many components and relates to many topics such as data mining, analytics, informatics, and AI. An in-depth discussion of these topics is outside the scope of this book, and each of them can be adapted into a book of its own. I will, however, point out how healthcare AIOps and ML cross-connect and that is that there is a need for ML to be the underlying technology in AIOps for the technology to work correctly.

NOTE   There is another concept to note, which is operations research (OR). OR is a "decision-tree" concept of AI where ML is the underlying science to create data for decision making, AI is the system that allows the decisions to be made in an automated way, and OR is considered the overlay to contrast with AI in that it is the decisions that are made with or without the automation. The "intelligence" part comes from the automation of actions, which we will cover in depth when we talk about the enterprise systems that allow AIOps to become a reality.

Now that you have a good understanding of AI, let's fuse this concept to healthcare. Healthcare is an ever-changing, evolving, dynamic field with many components. I like to divide healthcare into two separate realms when discussing AI: clinical and operational. These concepts were introduced earlier in the "Digital Transformation of Healthcare" section, and we will explore them further here.

Clinical AI is the use of AI, ML, and other intelligence components for clinical outcomes. As an example, if I want to trend what areas in a state are highest for the flu each year so I know where to stockpile medicine, I can data mine that information and make a clinical decision based on the results. This is the part of AI where ML allows us to use data mathematically to make decisions. Within the clinical realm, this use of AI and ML is still in its infancy, but major efforts are under way to develop innovative new technologies, tools, programs, systems, and workflows to more efficiently and effectively use clinical AI. Since this book focuses on the "operational" artificial intelligence realm, I will not delve too deeply into the clinical side except to make comparisons or show how clinical and operational AI at times will cross paths. However, it is important to know that AI in healthcare is very much a budding field where the positive clinical outcomes we seek and the innovation that is required to realize them is only just emerging.

AI in healthcare in the operational realm, or AIOps, is where most of our discussion in this book will focus. Operations can be defined as functions that keep the day-to-day business moving forward and ongoing. You can think of installing a server as a project where the management, maintenance, and patching of that server is the operational component needed to ensure the integrity of service. Not just healthcare, but all verticals, channels, fields, and roles require an operational component. Figure 1.1 shows the build-out of design, build, and run, which is a model that is commonly used to describe how we normally run an operation.

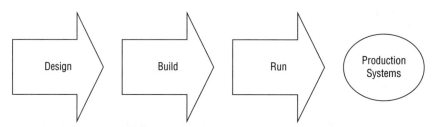

Figure 1.1: Design, build, and run model

The design, build, and run model is used when we want to do something like deploy a service (for example, a medical service like a new EMR system). First we design the service, then we build it, and then we run it.

The design phase is where we put together a strategy, create a project plan, procure funds, put a team together, and so on. The build phase is considered to be an engineering component to the workflow. We make something that needs to be managed or a service that needs to be maintained. At the end of the build process, the service is tested and, assuming it functions properly, is then signed off as production ready. Next, we run it. This is the operational component to the workflow. Now, it enters into monitoring systems so that it can be safeguarded from failure.

This is normal operational behavior for designing, building, and running anything, and in the healthcare space it is no different. However, there is one major difference to note that is a priority. The biggest difference that makes healthcare IT, healthcare operations, and other functions of healthcare service delivery more important than most other fields is that human lives are on the line. It is critical to keep in mind that there is a real "life or death" aspect to the things we do in healthcare. Therefore, when we monitor systems for use in a healthcare setting, having them operational and ready for use is an absolute top priority. This is where AIOps meets healthcare operations and helps to not only bolster that priority but act on it as designed.

USING ITIL IN HEALTHCARE OPERATIONS AND AIOps

Although this book is specifically about healthcare AIOps, being aware of how operations are generally built for the AIOps platform will help when you design and deploy your operations. One of the most widely used models that establishes IT best practices and guidance that you can use to deploy tools correctly is the information technology infrastructure library (ITIL). ITIL is a model used to help create a sound and reliable IT organization and is an important framework for modeling how to deploy reliable IT services. For example, there are five major sections to this model, which include service strategy, service design, service transition, service operations, and continuous process improvement. Each component of ITIL digs deeply into how a service is created all the way from inception through transmission and into production. It also creates an iterative function with continuous service review so that things can be improved especially as organizations and their services change. You can see an example of this in Figure 1.2.

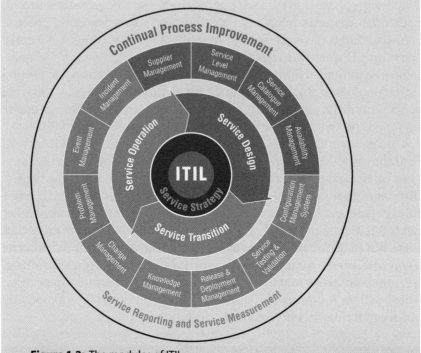

Figure 1.2: The modules of ITIL

The important takeaway here is that, as I noted with the design, build, and run model, services and systems need to be created well and managed in an ongoing and proper way so that they provide the required services. In healthcare operations, this becomes the fundamental factor of importance. When deploying AIOps, frameworks such as ITIL can help to ensure that once you get your services designed and deployed correctly, AIOps can deliver real value as an overlay and not just add confusion to poorly managed services that need some attention and focus.

Keep in mind that you can't build a good house on a weak foundation. Make sure that you consider the design suggestions listed in this section prior to your AIOps deployment to ensure that the house you build will be stronger and last longer.

Healthcare IT Operations

So, how does all of this fuse together to connect technology, healthcare, operations, and artificial intelligence? When you have a platform that can predict and respond, you have reached enlightenment. Today's operational systems usually lack interconnectivity and the ability to leverage the benefits of convergence. If we want to successfully navigate the roads of healthcare IT, we must build and pave them correctly. Only through proper planning and implementation will we deliver AI into healthcare IT operations.

The use of IT in healthcare is already deeply rooted and will continue to grow. Working in healthcare with paper files has been replaced with the EMR system and its interconnected world of computer technology that provides a clinical facility or doctor's practice more insight into how to provide care. Keeping that functionality up and running at all times can be complex and present an array of challenges. For example, if interconnectivity between systems is not operable, you may be missing components of the healthcare service you are trying to deliver. Let's look at some real-world scenarios where this might happen. If you want to get the results of bloodwork, you need the connection to the lab that processes that information, possibly with the proper credentials for security purposes. In another instance, if you want to prescribe medications, you need connections to the patient's preferred pharmacy (or the proper department if you're providing them within a hospital or other medical facility). In prescribing these medications, if your system has artificial intelligence that can check the patient's current medications and flag potential contraindications between them and your new prescription, that would be very helpful. To make such clinical decisions successfully and to the greatest benefit possible, you need the full, accurate data and functionality of all parts of the system.

Healthcare IT is the fundamental bedrock of allowing clinical services to operate with the technology that it deeply relies on in this day and age. HIT also contains elements of risk and the need for security, which is a critical part of HIT. That acknowledged, now let's consider how AI relates to HIT. AIOps is simply the fusion of HIT with AI that enables an enterprise system or service to take the data (such as that provided from ML and data mining) from production systems, learn patterns about ongoing production and day-to-day operations, and make predictions and decisions based on that data. For AIOps to function optimally in doing this, it needs to be mature, set up correctly, and given enough time to perform its tasks.

Applying AI to IT operations is one of the biggest benefits to healthcare operations as a whole. If we can deploy a system that can find our weak spots and either self-heal them or at minimum alert us to failure and make educated suggestions (or decisions) based on reliable data, we have evolved into the realm of enlightenment. This is one of the primary goals of all AIOps platforms. There is much that needs to be considered before we can realize that goal, and we will explore these considerations throughout this book. For the moment, I want to address fear.

There are many fears about this type of technology, and I will work to dispel any concerns with real-world experience on the subject whenever possible or share what other experts have uncovered in their strategizing and deployment of AIOps platforms in their environments. Most healthcare professionals' biggest fear would probably be, "If I deploy an AI solution that makes decisions without my approval, how would I know that those decisions are the right ones? What if a mistake is made?" Well, that is why this book will carefully examine all deployments of AIOps and how you can ensure that you are working with the best possible outcomes prior to and after deployment of these systems.

AI AND AIOps IN USE TODAY

Although this book will focus on enterprise platforms that deliver AI to manage large-scale operations, you should be aware of how hard and soft AI is used today all around you in healthcare, in IT, and in general. Today, everybody is delivering AI or AIOps. Every enterprise tool, platform, system, or application has the buzzword "AI" attached to it. The reason, quite simply, is that it sounds cool. More importantly, if we can achieve true AI, the benefits could be beneficial to us beyond our wildest dreams. But even the current state of AI is impressive. It is also pervasive. There are AI platforms in use today everywhere you look. Your mobile device, TV, and smart home device can connect to each other to use AI even more powerfully. Applications you use every day are AI functional. Obviously, the biggest ones are intelligent and can use functions like speech recognition such as Apple's SIRI, Google's Now/Home/Brain, Amazon's Alexa, Microsoft's Cortana, and others. Problem solving through decision trees can also be considered AI. Other platforms such as security systems, camera systems, and surveillance and monitoring systems can be automated to trigger alarms based on facial or other biometric information. There are so many others, too. Be aware that all of these functions have found their way into clinical operations and innovations as well as the HIT arena.

Healthcare AIOps functions can include technology we have already seen for years and is evolving into more AI-enabled platforms. These include IT technology such as antivirus (AV) platforms that use heuristics to make decisions on malicious software (malware) that can infiltrate your network and systems. For example, your AV platform can be loaded with a definition file so that it can analyze data and look for anomalies. This is one of the oldest forms of information technology and

AI from decades ago where you believed that your computer was smart because it could identify an attack pattern from a virus and quarantine it for you. The truth is, you had to keep those systems updated every single day (and you still do) with definitions that point the engines of the application to what those anomalies should look like. The heuristics function is the examination of that engine and the data that passes through it to make a "decision" or conduct an action based on that data. In mathematical terms, the heuristic function is making an intelligent decision based on information it knows to be right or wrong based on a threshold. As an example, an AV system might know that if it sees a high enough amount of a particular pattern on the system, that may be the sign of an attack, so the AV might send an alert to those who manage the system, flag the file as potential malware, or quarantine the file. This form of AI is the precursor for today's automated AI functions in a much larger world.

Another example of this type of technology is email spam filtering (based on rules), where if you flag something as spam, your email system will look at your email for patterns using data such as keywords, sender, Internet Protocol (IP) address, hostname, Domain Name System (DNS) server, and other technical qualifiers and automatically isolate those types of emails so you do not open them and spread a virus.

The same technology that local systems use for AV and spam filters can be seen in enterprise tool systems such as network-based intrusion detection and prevention systems (IDPSs) where the system captures data that traverses a network, recognizes potentially malicious anomalies, and blocks connections or quarantines data. The quarantining and blocking actions are considered the "intelligence" portion of the equation. However, you must remember that this information is acquired, learned, and ultimately refined at some point to identify outliers that do not match the proper patterns and might cause issues to the system if undetected. For example, you want to know if an email was erroneously flagged as spam and then quarantined when it actually should have been delivered. This requires tuning, refinement, and relearning. As we can see from systems of old, mistakes can be made just like in any other "intelligent" creature we know.

Figure 1.3 demonstrates this technology that AV systems, email spam filters, and IDPSs share. Basically, a heuristics engine keeps and updates a list of definition files that it can use to flag potential malware, scans data input for potential malware, and places malware in quarantine. This is one of the most common uses of AI in technology and the beginning of AIOps with security systems.

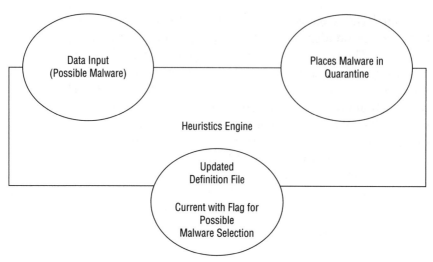

Figure 1.3: A heuristics engine using AI

Anything automated can be elevated to use AI. What truly makes it smart is that it has been configured to act that way. What makes it autonomous is its ability to do this without being told. You want to help your system become so smart that it borders on being autonomous so you can unlock its full power. Throughout this book, you'll see how to make smart, aware, and strategic decisions that allow you to benefit from this technology in the real world. When it comes to healthcare delivery, there can be no mistakes. Next we move into today's enterprise platforms that supply the AIOps experience to widescale systems and in a healthcare environment.

AIOps Platform Strategy

The impact of AI in health systems, EMRs, and other toolsets cannot be emphasized enough. Many AIOps platforms exist, but we will focus on the ones directly related to healthcare IT and how they can be leveraged to provide benefits to your enterprise architectures. Although we cannot cover them all, we will cover the most popular offerings. Before deploying an AIOps platform, your strategy has to be well thought out and executed with purpose. Make no mistake, purchasing this technology is expensive and will require approvals for budget dollars that may be questioned, so you need to select a great tool from a company that can back it with support, guidance, and documentation. You may require consulting fees and education credits for ongoing learning about the tool. You may need to educate a portion of your staff to operate and maintain the tools you purchase. Once you have selected a platform type, you will then need to know the players, options, services, functions, and offerings within that platform, and knowing the differences can make all the difference in your selection. Let's take a look at what those types are and how you can make a more informed decision on what you need for your strategy.

Platform Types

When considering AIOps platforms, it's important to know that just because something is called AIOps doesn't mean it's a plug-and-play tool that automatically learns everything on your network and makes great decisions. Quite the contrary. This is a complex environment that requires an understanding of the inner workings of service delivery, infrastructure, your core business, and all of its meticulous underpinnings. That said, let's break down some of these offerings so you are aware of how they differ and how they interconnect. In particular, we'll examine enterprise monitoring, information technology operations management (ITOM), and application performance monitoring (APM).

The first platform we'll examine is the enterprise monitoring and AIOps space. Tools are deployed enterprise-wide to encompass all architecture so that operational data can be ingested and learned and automation functions can be selected and applied based on patterns and trends that need to be considered. For example, Splunk (`splunk.com`) is an industry leader for AIOps and has been in business developing mature solutions for more than a decade. I will discuss Splunk further throughout this book. This type of platform can be on-site or cloud-based. The Splunk service can ingest data from connected systems and allow for high-level automated actions to take place. You can set up your network, servers, services, applications, systems, and other infrastructure on Splunk, and it will start to cross-examine the data to understand patterns between them to help you make educated decisions. When fully matured, Splunk can even be automated to make those decisions for you. An example may be that all of your network switches are performing poorly at and around 9 a.m. every workday for about 20 minutes. This trend is found to be caused by an excessive amount of access to a server farm located in your core network that is underperforming. You can be alerted to this issue so you can take action. Another futuristic model may show us being able to reroute traffic to a different server pool that is underutilized so that the load is more evenly dispersed.

Another platform type for AI is in the information technology operations management (ITOM)/information technology service management (ITSM) space. A leader in this space is ServiceNow (`servicenow.com`), another platform I will cover in depth in this book. ServiceNow is a service desk, service management, and, with ITOM, operations management platform that allows for incident triage, ticketing, asset management, and configuration management with configuration items (CIs), and ultimately it allows for AIOps through its platform. This is a more all-encompassing service management solution that performs different functions than a tool like Splunk, although Splunk may be a trusted source of data input into ServiceNow for ITOM.

Application performance monitoring (APM) is yet another platform to consider where AI is concerned. It is important to monitor and manage application performance. Although Splunk and ServiceNow offer similar functionality, an APM platform like Riverbed (`riverbed.com`) can be used to examine the end-user experience with the applications you deploy as services to them. APM will look at the services and how they perform based on AI via big data analysis it collects to make smart or automated decisions to help immediately solve customer problems.

So, as you can see, there is a myriad of offerings in different spaces. Enterprise monitoring, ITOM, and APM are the most sought-after solutions in healthcare IT and AIOps. However, other important platform choices exist, such as the ability to converge. So, as I noted before with ServiceNow, you may use this as your main ITSM tool with Splunk and Riverbed offerings added to complement infrastructure, applications, and other systems to create a complete package. Figure 1.4 shows how all of these systems (platforms) can be used together to offer one complete AIOps package in your enterprise.

Customer Experience and AIOps

All of technology is in place to make life easier, not the other way around. I know it seems to be the opposite sometimes, so we need to really focus on supplying solutions that benefit our customers in the end. When something is deployed into production, we should ask these questions: How did this help the company? Whom did it benefit in the organization? Did I get my return on investment (ROI)? Ultimately, how did this impact the customer? Ideally, the answers are positive ones.

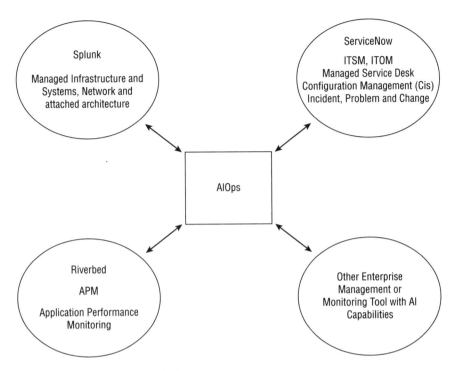

Figure 1.4: Convergence of platforms

Customer experience is the ultimate goal for all service offerings and solutions. All service delivery should be focused toward improving customer experience, and AIOps can help deliver a positive customer experience if done correctly. "Done correctly" is the key factor here. If you do not deploy these systems correctly, you never really get to the priceless benefits of full automation and decision making, and you therefore reduce your AIOps system to nothing more than a widely deployed and costly paperweight.

GETTING THE VALUE OF AIOps ON YOUR SYSTEM

Because AIOps is a pervasive overlay on your infrastructure, it impacts the performance of everything. When deciding how you want to use your AIOps platform, it is important to understand agent versus agentless technology. If you deploy an agent (an application or software program) to all systems you want to include in your AIOps deployment, it has to be considered as a possible impact to that system. We do not want to pay to deploy an AI system that does nothing more than just monitor for issues. We hope to deploy an AIOps platform that we can take full advantage of, which includes the learning, intelligence, and automated decision-making functions that make it so valuable.

AIOps Considerations and Goals

One of the biggest goals of AIOps is customer experience, but what does that translate to? For one, it means that when you use an AIOps solution, you will be able to improve your event correlation, incident triage, speed to root-cause analysis (RCA) with preventative and corrective actions, and automated decisions that can speed mean time to resolve (MTTR), which is a key metric when considering KPIs and CSFs. Key performance indicators (KPIs) and critical success factors (CSFs) are the holy grail of metrics to executives looking to ensure the ROI of deploying costly systems like AIOps. By focusing on the KPIs, you are well on your way to proving your AIOP's ROI. Figure 1.5 shows how these metrics are used to analyze and provide for better customer service.

Key Performance Indicator (KPI)	Explanation
Number of Repeated Incidents	Number of repeated incidents, with known resolution methods
Number of Incidents	Number of incidents registered by the service desk and grouped into categories
Average Initial Response Time	Average time taken between the time a user reports an Incident and the time that the service desk responds to that incident
Incident Resolution Time	Average time for resolving an incident and grouped into categories
Resolution within SLA (Service Level Agreement)	Rate of incidents resolved during solution times agreed in SLA

Figure 1.5: Analyzing KPIs for AIOps

Your second major goal should be transformation. By improving this triage, collection, handling, and resolving of problems (especially with automation), you are fundamentally transforming your workforce, technology environment, and overall footprint in the organization. Technology should always be recognized as a service. If it is not providing value, it is a detriment to the business and its ability to thrive. Technology needs to work for the business, not the other way around. By transforming your operations to be self-aware and actionable, you are raising the bar on transforming into the next age of technology offerings, operations, and service delivery.

Next should be innovation. If you are able to focus more on self-enlightenment of your technology, you will free time cycles to build on innovative solutions. As well, if your systems are fed with real-time data, you are able to make smart decisions on that data that should also help drive innovation. All of this in turn helps to create a better customer experience. Our customers include patients, clients, clinicians, business partners, and all the people we work and interact with, but they extend beyond that. Our customers include everyone who touches technology, which in this day and age is everyone.

Summary

In this chapter, we covered the fundamental knowledge needed to understand healthcare technology and operations as well as the fusion of AI to create AIOps. We covered a lot of important foundational information required to make smart decisions based on what tools you want to get, how to deploy them with a good strategy, and why they should be implemented in the first place. The focus of this introductory chapter was to begin your journey into the much larger word of AI and ML. AI and ML become increasingly important as the technologies around them have matured. We can now use AI and ML to help us reduce outages to our critical systems, improve interconnectivity, and perform other essential functions with growing confidence. This is where the importance of AIOps begins to emerge. I also touched on the importance of the EMR and its underlying infrastructure, how interconnected these systems really are, and how any impact to them could cause negative outcomes.

This chapter discussed the healthcare market and how technology has evolved, particularly within the AIOps space. AIOps is being used to create efficiency, reduce downtime, improve response time, reduce waste, and ultimately create a better experience for all patients, clinicians, and healthcare professionals. In the next chapter, we move beyond the foundational knowledge and dig deeper into AIOps and how to use it.

2

AI Healthcare Operations (Clinical)

*"Automation may be a good thing, but don't forget that
it began with Frankenstein."*

—**Anonymous**

As you strategize and deploy AI operations (AIOps) into your healthcare setting, you will want to immediately reap the benefits and rewards. What impact is made on the clinical side of the equation? As noted in the first chapter, there is no difference between AI and ML in their application to make things more adaptable and efficient; however, their benefits can be different based on what your goals are. In the clinical setting, our goals are to increase innovation and efficiency and allow for our data to be used in the best way possible to create better outcomes. AIOps can help this process by allowing for that data to be available, so in this chapter we delve into the clinical operations side of healthcare and how AIOps can provide for better outcomes aligned with clinical artificial intelligence applications.

This chapter discusses the use of AI, ML, and their applications in helping clinical operations, promoting innovation, streamlining, using big data, and providing for a better impact on informatics and analytics. In this chapter I explore more of the clinical side of AI and ML and why it's critical that we have an infrastructure that is reliable and secure.

The most important concepts to consider when discussing the clinical side of business operations is that IT (or technology) is used to augment and enable the abilities of the clinicians. I have heard two sides of this story where some believe that healthcare systems have become technology companies that do healthcare, and others believe that healthcare systems have invested heavily into technology departments so that more innovation can take place in the clinical realm. No matter what side you are on, the two now go hand in hand. Although we have the seamless delivery of care and service from our clinical leaders and teams, the use of technology becomes the vehicle in which it is now provided.

The two biggest takeaways from this chapter will be that AI and ML help us deliver care, and AIOps is the platform that makes that delivery possible.

Clinical Impact of AIOps

In today's setting, large companies such as Microsoft, Google, Apple, Amazon, and just about every other major technology company are placing large bets on artificial intelligence. It's also interesting to see how these companies are also getting into the healthcare space alongside AI and ML. For example, with Google, DNA collection and sequencing, identification, and use of big data are all the next steps for the company to grow its footprint into the future. All the major players have increasingly embraced AI and AIOps in a variety of ways. All the other smaller organizations have followed suit and are building out AI platforms and moving into the healthcare support space.

So, what about healthcare systems and providers? Where do they stand in all of this development? The first large-scale step in building big data solutions that can be used in clinical settings was to join forces and build large healthcare systems that could support these offerings. For example, most hospitals and practices have reached a place and time where to grow into the future of leveraging technology, joining a larger healthcare system is more of a requirement instead of an interest. That said, as more and more smaller systems join larger systems, the use and leveraging of tools (such as the ones I started to introduce) become possible. Once these steps have been taken, the real magic begins. Before I continue, I want to clarify the statement I just made on joining larger systems. Although not mandatory, hospitals, practices, providers, or health companies can join a larger healthcare provider or system to leverage assets. What I am pointing out is that to pay for large tools and technology that can be very costly, the joining of forces and sharing that cost become more palatable for those looking to use these tools and applications. Make no mistake, the use of AI, ML, and AIOps is a large-scale transformational change to how organizations will do business in the future, and more and more companies and businesses are getting involved. The more capital that exists to purchase these tools, start these projects, and conduct research and development (R&D), the more likely you are to scale up your clinical research and ability to conduct clinical innovations.

So now that you have an understanding of the importance of AI and ML on the clinical side of the business, what does AIOps bring to the table that becomes more of a need than a want? Many things. It begins with the forming of larger conglomerates in order to leverage technology and data to conduct intelligence operations and information analysis and ultimately identify trends in the data so it can be used in a positive way. An example in today's modern healthcare systems is the use of an entire health system's data trending to identify population health challenges such as "what diseases may be prevalent in certain areas." Without the collection and analysis of this data and its trends, we would not be able to make this prediction. Although this book does not fully focus on these types of trends and their outcomes, AIOps allows for clinical operations and analytics to become a reality.

The benefits of AIOps in the clinical space cannot be emphasized enough. You need a fully running, stable, and reliable technology operation that integrates all of the applications, databases, servers, networks, and other systems that collect, store, deliver, and process data from all of the different organizations that work together. This is essential for clinical operations and AI to exist and use the AIOps solutions in your technology operations space. That said, let's look at how both AIOps solutions and AI in the clinical space cross over to work symbiotically and create effective solutions.

TIP   Understanding how AI in the clinical space and AIOps solutions interrelate becomes increasingly important (and even crucial) to successful planning in the predeployment stages. Knowing what you plan to use the data for in the clinical setting allows you to deploy the appropriate technology to support it, which is foundational in real-world deployments.

Gaining a Competitive Edge with Intelligent Cloud, Data Analytics, and AI

Understanding how AI in the clinical space and AIOps interrelate becomes more and more important especially in the planning stages of the predeployment of these solutions. Cloud transformation in the healthcare space has revolutionized the ability to gather data, collect it on large databases, and conduct analytics and other AI operations to help drive predictive analytics. The use of AI and ML will allow for value growth beyond what the original datasets were intended for, and with cloud optimization, you are now able to grow the data flexibly (and cost effectively) while still allowing for innovation work to take place.

AIOps can use the combined capabilities of the cloud, analytics, and AI to ensure that all systems maintain high availability. This provides constant access to all data and the opportunity for using automation to act on any issues that are discovered. For example, if you are running a VMware solution to virtualize your server and database infrastructure hosted on virtual storage in the cloud, when any of these systems experiences an issue, the AIOps platform can step in and identify the issue, correct it, and allow for seamless operations to take place. This is where true fault and event management takes place to help reduce downtime. When you can automate these actions and create a self-healing workflow, you then make the system intelligent to help make decisions that can create that quick recovery time we would all desire. Think of a world where a healthcare system that had an application crash immediately resolved itself within minutes of happening. This would not only get clinicians back to work immediately, but also reduce the overhead and workload of the help desk by up to 90% based on the speed of self-healing.

Competitive edge can also be gained by using the cloud, particularly in the AIOps hosting opportunities the cloud provides. You can host your AIOps solution on-premise or in the cloud. A hybrid cloud solution can also be strategized for use if that fits your organizational needs. One thing that should be mentioned in the planning stages of using the cloud and AIOps is that security must be factored in so that any health information stored outside the walls of your healthcare facilities is safe and protected. Another big consideration is the solvency of the cloud provider and the contract stipulations, legal, and other compliance requirements that must be understood prior to putting data in the cloud. You will also want to ensure you have an exit strategy if needed to take your data outside the provider. Figure 2.1 shows the use of a cloud-based system with AI and AIOps.

Now that we have examined the foundational elements of AI and AIOps in a clinical space, let's explore the design and innovation considerations for your strategy to deployment, the challenges that lie ahead, where AIOps can enhance healthcare delivery, and service performance.

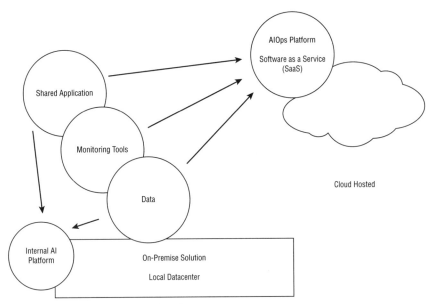

Figure 2.1: AI, AIOps, and the cloud

Design and Innovation

Design and innovation are two broad concepts. When planning design and innovation, one of the problems is that the planning can spiral out of control. As with any good planning session, you want to have clear boundaries of what you want to accomplish and, when you can, have a clear goal in mind. When brainstorming and considering the design of something or trying to create an innovation, you are trying to think outside the box, so it becomes a challenge to simultaneously keep the entire concept in perspective and zoom in to formalize clear steps and achievable goals. Sometimes we consider the use of SMART goals when looking to create a plan from our design sessions. This allows us to dream, but also to start grounded when it comes time to do work.

SMART GOALS

SMART goals are common in the business world today. SMART stands for specific, measurable, attainable, relevant, and time-bound. When you want to implement AI or ML tools in your environment, you will need a project plan, scope, and other planning criteria to make that a reality. You can use SMART goals when you begin the designing and brainstorming process.

An example would be that you want to allow for your health-based doctor directory to be automated and user-friendly so that when users log in, they can quickly pull a list of suggestions. The goal would be to design and deploy a search engine of health professionals that a patient could use to customize care based on the interaction between their current medical files and existing medical history. The index should be intelligent enough (or be able to learn well enough throughout this process) to make good suggestions to the patient as they search. The search function should be available in Q1 of next year to be deployed in the next cycle of upgrades.

In this example we can see that the goal is SMART in the following ways:

■ The goal is specific and so is the outcome (design and deploy a search engine).

■ The goal is also measurable. You can see from the output and other metrics pulled if the results come back in a way that creates value.

■ The goal is attainable because you have the technology in place to do this project and have approval to move forward.

■ The goal is relevant because it is a needed service that will add value to the patient experience.

■ The goal is time bound because you set a specific amount of time in which you wanted to achieve the goal.

Use SMART goals to help develop your efforts in a way where you can strategize your next steps without waste.

The business of health delivery is a large, complex, and all-encompassing operation. One of the key components of moving into a world of AI and ML is design. Design can be thought of as planning, strategy, foundation, and pre-development work. In simple terms, if you wanted to build a house, you would consider deploying the foundation that can support the house prior to doing any work on the house at all. The same concepts need to be applied to the consideration of using AI of any kind in an organization. To the experts, AI becomes the overlay that we would apply to all of the foundational items that would be firmly in place prior to deploying it. Consider the technology needed to provide informatics teams with their data. The data can be mined from databases that are housed in data warehouses, and when considering big data scenarios, they are likely housed on large-scale, high-speed storage platforms that are redundant and resilient. When these items are in place, then and only then would an AIOps platform be helpful.

Another consideration is the "all or nothing" rule in deploying an AIOps platform. When you want to design for automation and real machine learning scenarios where actions are reported and then taken through intelligent systems, how can those decisions be made if you have bad data in place? Would that mean that bad decisions would be made? Or, what if you wanted to have a self-healing system where the action would be to reboot the system and because of bad data, false positives existed and you rebooted a server providing services to clinical systems that was not having an issue? This is why true AIOps systems need to be designed and built in a foundationally firm environment where good data can be used to make good decisions.

TIP   Another important foundational element to be used as a building block with developing an AIOps platform strategy is to have a solid IT asset management (ITAM) solution in place with a configuration management database (CMDB) that can be leveraged as a source of truth on identifying the systems, assets, and services in your ITSM portfolio.

The use of asset control, configuration items (CIs), and CMDB will allow you to create a single source of truth (SSOT) for your overlaid systems. An SSOT is a way of ensuring that all data is managed in one place, and all other parties refer to the data through that source. What this means is if you decide to deploy a service management solution or tool that requires the use of your company's information, such as servers, system types, IP address ranges, site locations, and the myriad of other data that any platform would need, having that in a master data set would be the foundational item required for any major deployment to be more successful. Make sure you consider ITAM, CMDB, and other trusted sources prior to any major management or monitoring tool deployment like AIOps.

Once the design has been achieved, then innovation can be considered. Innovation in this context can be the AIOps platform itself and how you plan on deploying it so that it can take whichever actions you want. So, when we consider artificial intelligence as the way forward to innovatively take actions, create activities, and produce functions that mimic human intelligence, one would think that selecting the right AIOps platform would be a foundational item based on what functionality you want to plan for. You may want to mimic robotic actions based on intelligence learned and actions taken through automation so that the storage platform your data is hosted on is self-healing. That would mean that the innovative design approach would take the storage array design approach first with the AIOps platform as the overlay. In this scenario, I may want to create a design that looks similar to Figure 2.2, where the storage array is laid out in a physically redundant fashion, where each array has redundant drives, and the drive arrays themselves are virtualized, snapshotted, and placed redundantly offsite if needed. All database servers are loaded onto virtualized machines (VMs), and the system is also redundant and self-healing. The logic between the databases is also redundant, and each database node is set up in a cluster with a dedicated data quorum and protected transaction log. From there, the entire system is duplicated and replicated off-site to a secondary site that can be used if the original site is impacted.

Now, your foundational items for this particular system design are covered. You can next overlay your agents or system interfaces for your AIOps platform to manage, monitor, alert, and react to operational issues as they occur. For example, if your AIOps platform is installed correctly and has had time to learn, it should be able to provide automation in the sense that if you get a triggered alert from a failed part of the system, the platform should be able to help it self-heal without any human interaction at all. In a true machine learning environment, the ability for the technology to learn without being specifically programmed could provide a response to the failure. For an AI solution, the preprogrammed responses can be taken based on time spent learning the system's baselines and knowing that something is taking place outside the normal thresholds and is considered an anomaly. This anomaly may have a preprogrammed action that needs to take place, such as fail over database server node A to node B if node A is no longer responsive to data requests.

It is my goal to ensure that before you begin down the road of deploying an AIOps solution, you are 100% aware of what is required prior to doing so. Now, let's take a quick look at what could happen if design and innovation are not considered as foundational items. For some, it may be tempting to install an AIOps platform into their environments believing (or maybe not believing) that they are ready to do so. For example, if your storage platforms were not redundant, if your database nodes had problems properly failing over, if issues were causing failovers that were false positives or worse, if your redundant drives were failing and an action was taken to fail over to a failed disk, and so on, we can see how "automated" actions (based on machine learning or otherwise) could create more problems than the original one that may have surfaced.

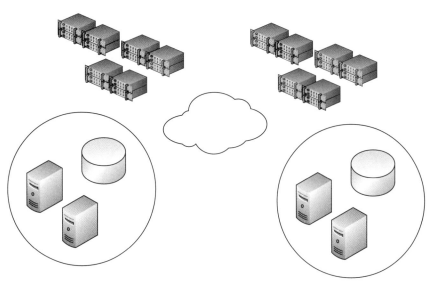

Figure 2.2: Redundancy in the system

> **CAUTION**   The design and consideration of the tools you deploy can profoundly benefit or impact your ability to deliver healthcare as a service. AIOps platforms are expensive. You will want to get ROI for your money spent, so you need to make sure you deploy AIOps correctly. Clinical systems can benefit from AI, but they can also be impacted by a bad deployment. Consider the scenario in a clinical operation where we collect a massive amount of data to try to cure a disease and, in that collected data, we mess up and collect a large amount of data on three different diseases, losing focus on the one we intended to work with. The data from the one particular disease would be mired with bad information, which would cause the data to be useless. This is the same thing with AIOps. If you do not deploy it correctly, it will not tell you what you need to know, and if you deploy the automation portions to take action, actions taken on bad data can be catastrophic to your operation.

AIOps for Healthcare Delivery

Healthcare delivery is exactly what it sounds like—the delivery of healthcare to a population from a healthcare system and providers. Healthcare delivery is another extremely broad term that needs to be drilled down into so we can better understand why it's critical to healthcare systems and how AIOps can benefit it or impact it. What does a healthcare delivery system look like? Figure 2.3 shows a small window into a larger world of healthcare delivery but gives you enough insight so that you can understand the scope of what an AI system or AIOps platform must encompass once deployed.

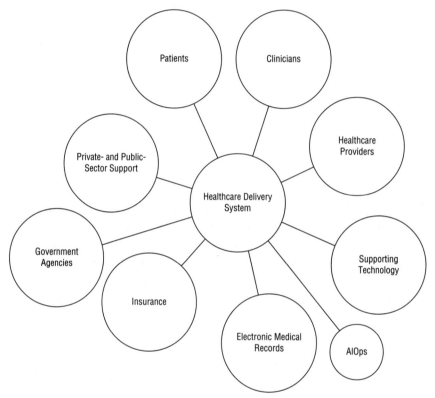

Figure 2.3: Healthcare delivery connects many people and systems.

The benefits of using an AIOps platform for healthcare delivery are numerous. The first and most obvious one would be that a correctly deployed and functional AIOps platform allows you to streamline your business. The best way to explain what streamline means is to consider wasted time. If your human assets are spent doing basic tasks that can be automated and you implement AIOps, these same assets can then move on to doing more strategic work, planning, deployment, and process improvement work, just to name a few.

WARNING   One of the biggest challenges in recommending, designing, deploying, and maintaining an AIOps platform is the human element.

Humans believe that artificial intelligence will take their jobs and leave them unemployed. One of the tactics I have used personally in this situation is skill enhancement and relearning. The deployment of AIOps is similar to how the cloud became a disruptor. Those who ran the systems in local data centers became new support staff and business liaisons between their organization and the cloud service provider. In the same way, someone needs to automate, program, manage, monitor, and maintain tasks and the AIOps platform. New skills will be needed, but more importantly, the institutional knowledge of the existing workforce needs to be preserved for helping devise strategy and automation processes for the platform. There is no need to replace people. Instead, the need is to augment their existing skills with new ones. If anything, as long as you explain to your current employees how the new platform will benefit not only the company but also the workforce, you will have a strategy for deploying the AIOps platform with minimal disruption from the people who will transition to maintaining it.

Healthcare delivery requires technology, and technology needs to be maintained and managed. AIOps provides the enterprise toolset that allows you to manage and monitor (and react to) all operational issues taking place that could disrupt healthcare delivery. Let's look at another example (Figure 2.4) of how the disruption of an EMR could shut down an entire hospital system and how AIOps if strategized and deployed properly could help with this use case.

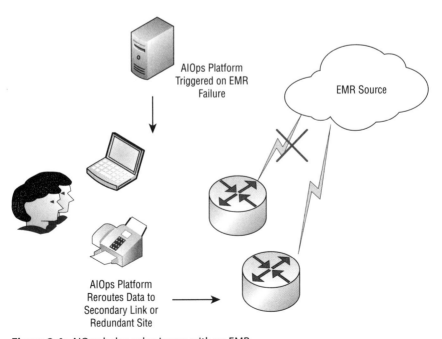

Figure 2.4: AIOps helps solve issues with an EMR.

Using AIOps in healthcare from a clinical perspective can really help make the case for a purchase and deployment opportunity. In this example, we had an entire healthcare-providing facility or hospital completely disrupted. Everyone had to go to downtime procedures (filling in old-fashioned paper forms that later needed to be uploaded into the system which is twice the work) to have a continuity of operations (COOP) event. In this situation, the EMR platform was unable to take notes from doctors because of a failed module or service within the system. When this first happened, the only way it was identified was when the doctors and other clinical staff had to stop what they were doing (providing care) to call the help desk or log on to open a ticket and file a complaint. When the help desk became aware of the issue, they began to triage it. They determined that several different calls also came from other providers who were experiencing the same issue, which alerted everyone to the fact that it could be a global issue with the EMR and not localized to the first hospital that reported it.

Once the issue was recognized as global, priorities were escalated, and incident teams and application teams then met on call bridges and war rooms to work on identifying and isolating the issue's root cause. While this testing was taking place, doctors were hand-writing prescriptions, instructions, and various notes. Patients also needed to be consulted or given medication, requiring the doctor's existing notes to be used and new information to also be written. At this time, perhaps 45 minutes to an hour of downtime had elapsed, and in a good scenario, the application teams were able to identify the root cause and how to fix it. The change management team was then consulted, and the application teams implemented the fix. The system was then stabilized, and when time allowed, the clinicians updated all their handwritten data into the EMR.

This same example can be used for scans, X-rays, blood draws, medications, and the list goes on and on. As you can see, any disruption at all not only can cause a disruption in care, but it can also invite errors, which is also highly problematic and concerning. So, what does an AIOps platform bring to the table to help healthcare delivery? For one thing, it absolutely drives down the mean time to resolve (MTTR), which is a valuable key performance indicator (KPI) and critical success factor (CSF)—metrics that help to show executives and those below them that the work they do, the purchases they make, and the plans they enact actually provide benefits. In the use case scenario with the EMR, the next biggest gain would be that we could identify the root cause and streamline problem analysis with corrective and preventative actions (CA/PA), which are ITIL basics for service operations (SO) and problem management (PM).

Incident management (IM) is also greatly benefited with AIOps because that MTTR can be addressed, but also the problem resolution in tandem, which allows the help desk to be alerted as the systems are alerting them, and this usually happens through an operations center (typically referred to as a NOC). If the AIOps platform identifies that the connection from one server to another has been impacted causing the "notes" function to not be connected to the EMR, it can then alert the operators at the NOC that this has a cause and effect. The "learning" portion of ML and AI in this scenario can then report on, if viewed, that this same scenario has happened 22 times in the past calendar year and that the same solutions were put in place, which was a "restart of the service."

Two important facts are exposed at this time about this use case. First, there was a preventative action put in place, not a corrective one, in the root-cause analysis (RCA) of the previous failures. Second, the restarting of a service is a preventative measure if and only if it's done prior to the failure in hopes to prevent it, or it becomes a corrective action if it's done to regain service. However, the restarting of a service doesn't truly correct the failure if it's recurring. Because of this, the AIOps platform would "learn" that this is a common occurrence and could be programmed with logic to restart the service at period intervals until the application team and application vendor or provider could implement a fix (perhaps a bug patch or logic programming change). However, until then, the intelligence of the system has kept the service up and running without failure. This is but one of hundreds of ways that the AIOps platform can provide an ROI based on downtime, costs, and patient impact, which can cause a reputation issue. The automated correction of issues can be as simple as a service restart. The system can be more elaborate and reboot servers, send data down different network paths, and on and on. This leads to better decision making, better reporting, and better identification of problems that need to be looked into and resolved outside the AIOps platform.

NOTE   One of the benefits of AIOps and healthcare delivery is that you are given the tools and a dashboard (most AIOps platforms have them) to do advanced reporting and metrics. When you can work from data-driven business information, insights, visualizations, and graphs, and plug that data into enterprise tool sets to do predictive analysis, you can be better at design, strategy, planning, and decision making, which brings us full circle to our foundational concepts of design and innovation.

AIOps for Service Performance

Using healthcare AIOps for service can improve your service performance metrics, which are also critical for reporting. Healthcare challenges and the need for AIOps will only grow exponentially as the systems we use become more complicated.

Think of it this way: how far have we come with technology since 1990? Then consider where we were 10 years ago when healthcare in America was in need of an overhaul and EMRs needed to be deployed, compliance needed to be met, and systems needed to be integrated. We are infants in this space with a long way to go to maturity, but fortunately technology allows us to grow quickly. However, we need to be smart with how we deploy and use that technology so we can reap its true benefits and not just waste time and money on failed projects and efforts. For example, we can use a dashboard to look at service performance, report on how each service rates with a scorecard, and know how the AIOps platform was able to keep services successfully running and restore them when necessary. This is how we as leaders can justify purchasing, licensing, and upkeep of million-dollar, large-scale platforms.

Service performance scorecards are critical for internal leaders to review how they are performing but even more critical to show a vendor how they are performing and whether they are violating service-level agreements (SLAs) or service-level objectives (SLOs), which could be punishable by monetary fine. Figure 2.5 shows software tracking performance metrics.

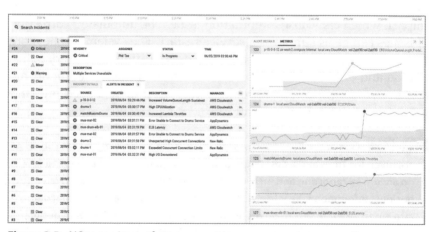

Figure 2.5: AIOps service performance metrics

The target for these metrics is consistency with trends that are under-stood. In the example shown in Figure 2.5, the service seemed to be highly disrupted in the months of June and July. We can identify what outages, errors, actions, and triggers occurred and get a better idea of the service impact so we can determine a reason for the disruption. In this example, an answer was found. The problem was that during the time noted, a major upgrade of the vendor's application caused disruption because new software updates were not tested well and caused issues until they were replaced (in late July), which stabilized the system. The metrics of service performance, scorecards, and data reports were able to show the leadership team that the vendor or application teams needed to do a better job of testing and validating the system prior to deployment. The AIOps platform was able to provide this data and thus justify its value to the organization.

In the future, as systems become more complicated, the use of AIOps platforms will be mandatory. We will be challenged to keep up with the growth, staffing needs, and financial costs of technology. We will also need to demonstrate the improved performance and financial benefits that the AIOps platform provides to our organizations. The metrics provided help to bolster the argument for the continued deployment of AIOps so that more automation can take place to identify and resolve problems.

Now that we have identified why AIOps is critical for the success of clinical operations, we are going to discuss the importance of clinical AI, healthcare information, and analytics, and how they will ultimately converge with AIOps in a future where all systems will be interconnected and share data for better outcomes.

Clinical AI, AIOps, and Future Platform Convergence

In the past five years, AI has evolved radically and will continue to do so far beyond what it is today. The involvement, integration, and convergence of AI platforms will experience increasing attention as we move into the future. Before we explore the point of convergence, let's take a look at the other side of the coin when it comes to clinical AI and healthcare.

Data collection in healthcare systems can be a convoluted process, and those who seek care do not really see its benefits in today's healthcare world. For example, right now I am positive that everyone reading this book has gone to receive care (or knows someone who has) and has had to provide the same information over and over again every time they visit a specialist, provider, clinician, doctor, nurse, or other care provider. Some of the information needs to be duplicated, like height, weight, and other vitals that are taken every time and entered into the EMR system. However, reporting if you have ever had diabetes is probably something that they can pull from the EMR themselves. The point is, there are a lot of gaps in the data collection process in clinical healthcare right now, which is something that the healthcare systems are focused on fixing. Ensuring that our data collection process works as well as possible is crucial because it is essentially what comprises big data, which healthcare informatics depends on. Healthcare informatics uses this collected data to deliver healthcare, provide healthcare services, and provide clinical service to our patients.

You can converge big data, informatics, AIOps, and ML, and then do the overlays with tools and toolsets. The convergence then comes in the form of innovation where all of these systems interact with each other to provide efficiency through automation.

One more use case we can look at with healthcare delivery and convergence could be retrieved from our earlier examples. In the example in which the EMR was not able to collect notes from doctors, which impacted service, the application was housed on the storage system and supplied via the database that was impacted. The convergence of big data and informatics is when we cannot provide good predictive analytics on notes collected from Type 1 diabetes patients who use insulin regularly and become resistant to it. Figure 2.6 shows how all of these systems feed into the analytics used by a clinician trying to make a diagnosis or an informatics analyst looking to understand the data to find a trend and make a suggestion or prediction. If you impact these systems, you impact the workflow.

Using big data to find opportunities is one of the primary goals of AI. If the system that supplies the clinician with the ability to provide care is down and impacted, how can that information be used correctly to predict outcomes or find trends? If systems are not able to run properly and cause corruption to the data we rely on, how can we trust that the data is accurate and usable? How AI and ML help to deliver better outcomes in healthcare is simple—it's the combined efforts of all platforms, tools, technologies, and analysis that when applied together create a real use for the collected data that can be leveraged and analyzed to produce benefits and results.

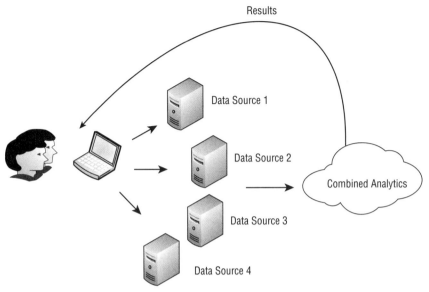

Figure 2.6: AI converged

Security and Privacy

Now we will explore the importance of security in AI, technology, and healthcare in general. To put it simply, we as technologists, healthcare providers, or anyone working with or in the healthcare space have a legal, moral, and ethical responsibility to protect the data of our patients at all costs. There is no excuse for not doing so, and the penalties can be high. Not only can it impact your career as a healthcare worker, but it can impact the lives of those you jeopardized.

Why Security Is Paramount in AIOps

Put yourself in the shoes of others to help better understand the risks or impact of decisions you may make when it comes to healthcare technology and systems. You are collecting the data of everyone who comes into the healthcare system for care. This data collectively represents entire communities, cities, and states, but it represents each individual as well. Just about everyone in the world who has access to healthcare uses data, and their individual data is private to them and them alone.

The only people privy to this information are those who are entrusted to keep it private, which is anyone working in the healthcare environment.

PHI, HIPAA, and other healthcare security standards are in place to protect the privacy of those we must protect. Although I will break each of these down momentarily, it must be stated that all of these security laws, compliance, systems, features, and so on cannot really protect the privacy of those around us; it really comes down to us as individuals. For example, say you are an ER nurse and you see someone famous come in for what may be an embarrassing reason. It may be life threatening. It could be damaging to their career. Whether someone is famous or not (I just used that as a dramatic example to make a point), everyone deserves the same treatment when it comes to privacy of data.

All healthcare security standards work to protect data, privacy, and confidentiality and together provide a framework that can be followed when using a system or platform. Collectively, they help to guide your security policy and ensure that you constantly secure data and monitor, test, and improve your security, as shown in Figure 2.7.

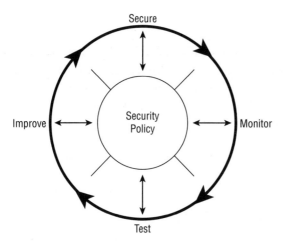

Figure 2.7: AI security framework

With AIOps (or any AI system in general), you need to make sure you are compliant with the security advice provided by your healthcare system that you work for or with, or consult for. You are responsible, and that must be fully understood. As you work with big data, data collection, and the possibility of having access to private information, you need to make every effort to realize that protected health information (PHI) is your responsibility to safeguard.

HIPAA, PHI, and PII Protection

Protected health information is part of the Health Insurance Portability and Accountability Act (HIPAA), which in 2003 was put in place as a US law to protect the privacy of patients, their medical records, and other personally identifiable health information. When people violate HIPAA, it can cause massive fines, penalties, and problems for healthcare systems. It also means that someone could be held personally responsible and even be terminated from employment.

Because of that, it is important to know that when working with big data, AI, and other sources of information, you need to remain vigilant and protect it. You cannot send the information in an email unprotected to others. You cannot access data files and folders that contain information you should not see. If you gain access, you need to not go where you are not allowed to go. You must always be careful and aware.

Personally identifiable information (PII) is different than PHI; however, it can also be damaging, so it needs to be treated with privacy as well when it comes to its use. When collecting and using data, information that can personally identify someone has to be redacted so that it cannot be used as part of the analytics performed. Someone's name is not important, but if they had the flu and lived in New York, got their flu shot in a specific year, were 72 years old, were male or female, or died from the flu is important. As I noted, making clinical predictions requires all of this but does not require someone's name.

So, how does AI, ML, and AIOps connect to the security framework, and how do we make sure we remain secure? If in doubt, consider privacy over a careless mistake. Situational awareness is important in this area. You have to consider that any data you collect could be sensitive and must be protected. AI for clinical settings absolutely keeps private information intact, and you need to consider that at all times, but what about AIOps data?

WARNING   As we move into the future of data collection and analysis, remember that biometric data is now collected and can be used. DNA data is collected and can be used. All of this must be identified as private and protected at all costs.

AIOps data must remain secure, and it is the main reason why all of the technology systems that house the data that you are protecting must also remain protected. If someone is able to access an AIOps system, they may gain access to information that can exploit the systems that contain patient data and provide a way to expose it. All systems must remain confidential and secure. One leads to the other and can affect exposure.

Another way that exposure can be affected is based on how encompassing your AIOps platform is. For example, if you are collecting data for your security systems or communication systems, you may have ingress and egress filters collecting data or blocking it, which can have repercussions when someone sends an email with PHI and the email filtering system captures and quarantines it. You may be able to access that because the AIOps system identified it. As already noted, one leads to the other, and vice versa, so in the spirit of convergence, remain vigilant on all fronts and we can continue a high level of security, privacy, and confidentiality of patient data no matter what service we work on in the healthcare system.

AIOps AND SECURITY

Being able to accurately provide detection of threats is one of the biggest gains for any security team in any enterprise. If a malware exposure takes place, there is a penetration, or there is some form of data breach or theft, the ability to get ahead of it (or know about it at all) is paramount to the future organization's survival. Some of the ways AIOps can bring immediate benefits to your security infrastructure is in the way of analyzing these threats in real time and, in some cases, immediately handling them. For example, AI in network access control (NAC) is for the quarantining of any device that joins the network without updated antivirus (AV) signatures. AIOps can overlay this by not only alerting to it but taking other actions on top of it so that perhaps more logic can be applied to apply the updated signature or replace the system with a new image (as examples).

The following are other benefits:

- Threat detection
- Threat remediation
- Quarantining
- Replacement

As we move into the next few chapters, we will focus on topics such as security so you are aware of what benefits you can get with the AIOps platform in securing your assets.

Lastly, another area to consider is the security of financial data. The Payment Card Industry Data Security Standard (PCI DSS) and the systems that interconnect to provide security for those paying for healthcare services must also be protected. Security may be monitored as part of the cardholder data environment (CDE) that may also be integrated with the AIOps platform, so making automation choices, keeping personal information private, and knowing how to quickly solve problems also become important when we consider security.

Summary

This chapter focused on the clinical aspects of AI and ML and how they blend into the use of AIOps. To make this crystal clear, you can have the clinical side of big data, informatics, and analytics to conduct research, trending, forecasting, enhanced patient care and services, as well as improved healthcare delivery, but you can keep all of that up and running with little impact with an AIOps systems management and monitoring solution. As we will see in the future and with larger health systems growing big data sets and sharing them within and throughout used toolsets, we may find that a trusted data source can serve both the clinical as well as the operational system of healthcare.

AI Healthcare Operations (Operational Infrastructure)

"Hope is not a strategy."
—Vince Lombardi

As you strategize and deploy AI operations (AIOps) systems into your healthcare setting, you will want to make an impact on your operational management and monitoring of critical systems that keep your health system running and optimized for clinicians, patients, and other users who are dependent on its availability. The goal will be to first design and then deploy an AI platform that can be used to its maximum potential. An AI platform that is deployed correctly will allow for automation or tasks that will help to keep your systems running when different issues appear.

This chapter discusses the knowledge you must have to not only plan but also prepare for an AI operations platform that is appropriate for your organization. This chapter will explore some of the current products on the market. However, you can replace any of the products listed here with newer or alternate solutions because the key concepts remain the same—you cannot build a house on a weak foundation and expect the house to remain standing especially in times of crisis. Once the system is designed, deployed, and operational, you have to make sure that it's used to its full extent so that the true benefits of AIOps can be explored and gained.

Getting Started with AIOps

Using AI in healthcare operations provides many benefits. The importance of keeping critical systems operational so that healthcare operations can run and continue to run during any technology issue is the primary benefit of using AIOps platforms in a healthcare environment. Technology that keeps your electronic medical records (EMRs) available, labs running, operating rooms operating, and emergency departments triaging patients without any loss of time due to an outage is every healthcare system's goal. To turn this goal into a reality, we must focus our strategy appropriately.

In today's modern technological healthcare system–driven operations, the use of technology is no longer optional. Any outage of the infrastructure, applications, systems, or services that supply clinicians with their tools cripples their ability to perform at a high-performance rate. Our goal should be to keep the clinical staff conducting clinical operations while those who run the administrative backend, such as providing needed technology, should focus primarily on keeping those tools operational and available. This is where designing an AIOps strategy starts to take shape.

ESTABLISHING YOUR ROI

When proposing or recommending the costly purchase of an AIOps platform for your organization, you should cover the following in your proposal statement:

- Reducing impact on clinical operations through the use of technology that allows immediate identification of issues

- Identifying the root cause and providing its solution in a fully developed system

- Using automation that allows for the healing of those issues as they occur

Doing these things will reduce your overhead, and your return on investment (ROI) will be realized in the future with a reduced impact to systems that provide services and a reduced footprint on maintaining disjointed systems that do event monitoring and management. The ultimate goal will be to provide automation that allows for self-healing when appropriate, which will help to reduce the mean time for resolving an issue from an outage, which is a KPI most executives are interested in hearing about in technology-driven companies.

Now that you have decided to implement an AIOps platform for your organization, your first step should be to determine your strategy and design for deploying it based on your goals. For example, if one of your goals is to reduce outage time and increase recovery time for failed technology assets, then you want an AIOps platform that can help you accomplish this. The term used to define the goals you want to achieve based on the solutions you will deploy is a *use case*.

With AIOps, use cases are part of every marketing kit that comes as a standard with any product you investigate. Most of them address the same issues that are present in most organizations today. Here is a list of common use case scenarios and the verbiage associated with them from a marketing perspective:

- There is a need to reduce the time involved with silos in organizations when trying to support an issue.

- There is a need to move from theory to practice to reality.

- There is a need to solve challenges that span the organization using automation and self-healing technology.

- Have technology work for you through the use of correct product selection and deployment.

- AIOps is transformative and will take your organization to the next level.

- Solve issues with reputation by managing issues quicker to resolution with AIOps.

- IT operations teams are normally disjointed, not allowing for the quick and expedient resolution of issues.

- To prevent, identify, and resolve high-severity outages and other IT operations problems more quickly, businesses are turning to artificial intelligence for IT operations.

- There is a need for advanced event management and analysis that allows the use of one platform to automate workflow and corrective actions.

- There is a need for noise reduction within your organization's operational realm.

- Root-cause analysis (RCA) and determination are required for service management maturity.

- Creating thresholds, triggers, and alarms that are actionable will allow for your system's issues to be corrected more quickly.

- Anomaly detection (outliers) will outshine the trends that AIOps identifies.

- Predictive analytics will help to promote a more stable environment by using the data gathered and identified by AIOps to provide high-level service intelligence.

Use cases are important to developing strategy, and it's likely that if you are shopping for a product, some form of the content I just listed is either something you are thinking of using AIOps for or something that the product vendor is telling you the system architecture will do for you. Buyer beware, not all of this can be solved by deploying AIOps software. There will be cases where only when you deploy all of the tools offered and let them run in your environment problem free for a period of time (such as three months), where baselines can be established and automation can be configured, will some of these use case items become reality. This is not meant to discourage you but set expectations and empower you to have the correct conversations with your internal stakeholders as well as with the product vendors who want to make a sale.

Strategy of AIOps Deployments

Some of the greatest developments of technology in the past decade include artificial intelligence, machine learning, and the fusion of technology and healthcare so that clinical outcomes can be better, more efficient, and dependable. All of these concepts sound great, but deploying them requires a sound strategy. There is a lot of talk around AI and not enough action. There are a lot of products on the market today that promise to deliver results, but in reality, if used incorrectly, they will actually cause more problems and deliver very little in the way of actionable solutions for the cost, time, and investment needed to deploy them.

To fully understand the benefits and put them in practice, you must strategize how AI will in fact change your IT operations and infrastructure services for the better with the addition of the AIOps service. By correlating real-time events with automation of responses to help minimize disruptions in critical IT functions in healthcare organizations, the AIOps platform, systems, and services will create an overlay that promotes self-healing.

You should start your strategy by doing an assessment of all the infrastructure you would like to maintain in the AIOps system and the outcomes you would like to get once you have deployed it. A simple goal statement could be to manage, monitor, and create automated actions for reducing mean time to resolution (MTTR) for critical systems that support the healthcare system's EMR platform. The systems that host and support an EMR platform include Windows, Linux, IBM, Citrix, VMware, and EMC storage platforms as well as all interconnected Cisco network devices. Once all systems are incorporated into the AIOps platform, two to three months of collected data will be analyzed and reviewed for areas of improvement that can be gained from automation provided by the AIOps platform.

Once you can express a high-level goal statement, you can then drill down into each segment of the goal statement and define what each of these sections will look like once completed. This can help you create a scope and define what your costs and resources will be not only to roll out the initial base system, but to maintain it and realize its benefits. These large-scale systems are not plug and play. They require agents on systems or configurations to be made that need access to and have the ability to modify production systems.

Creating a Scope

Once you have established your strategy, your next steps should be to create a scope statement and assess what products you may like to use from the myriad of vendors available. A statement of work (SOW) should be put together using basic project management principles. The SOW allows you to understand that whatever you "scope" your project to look like is what you will deploy when the time comes. This is important because you need to develop a budget that will provide the capital for your initial purchase and the ongoing operating expenses. When developing a scope, you can use Figure 3.1 for a general framework of what you will need to follow to get through the rest of the project phases. You will need to strategize what the project will look like and what resources will be needed. (Resources can be monetary as well as human.) You will then move through your deployment until completion. Once this phase is completed, monitoring, support, maintenance, upgrades, and overall management of the product will continue through the product's lifecycle. From there, adjustments will be made, especially as the product changes and your organization changes (size, function, role), and then you go back to strategize how you need to deploy or redeploy your system.

This general overview should help you understand your current environment and conceptualize your deployment so you can select the best vendors for your needs.

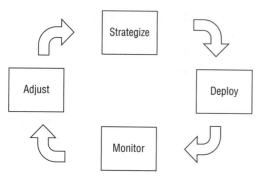

Figure 3.1: Reviewing a scope of work

Understanding that one size doesn't fit all is also an important part of scoping your project. You may find after doing some analysis that you may have to deploy your AIOps platform in stages over time. You may find that you have other AI systems in your organization that may work well with the AIOps platform you may want to deploy or, quite the opposite, that it may require a large amount of configuration and management to get them all to work correctly. This will all be worked out in the initial proof of concept (POC), or the pilot phase, so that you can see what works well (and what doesn't) with your environment while attempting to meet your proposed goal statement.

NOTE *POC* and *pilot* are two closely related terms. POC is basically the testing of the feasibility of a project to determine how well it will work. When trying out an AIOps platform, some of this can be accomplished through researching how well the product works in the market, and some of it can be accomplished by running tests within your organization and getting feedback from stakeholders. This also helps mitigate risk both during initial implementation and down the road. A pilot is basically the initial rollout of the product for the purposes of testing it, which can also be done as part of the POC.

NOTE Chapter 4 will discuss in more depth the specifics of an actual project, project plan, resource requirements, and an expanded scope. However, we're touching on these concepts here to help you with your goal statement and basic scope of work. Understanding this information before doing a proof of concept, pilot, vendor selection, or any other product review will save you time so you can focus on what you need to get the goals accomplished and within budget.

Strategy also puts a spotlight on selection considerations and designing healthcare AIOps systems to fit your needs and also create an impact based on ROI. You will be tempted by what you hear in marketing proposals by vendors, but make no mistake, it doesn't always work as intended or reported. Mixed and hybrid systems, such as cloud and internal system mixed architecture, cause challenges where you may not be able to deploy agents on systems within a cloud provider. You may not be able to set up connectors. You may have mixed systems (vendors) as well, which causes challenges such as mixing a tool like Splunk with a Cisco management tool, a Windows management tool, and a Citrix management tool. They may not snap together perfectly and may require some adjustments and additional customization. Also pay close attention to supported and nonsupported systems, such as open and closed architecture, which may also create challenges to your deployment. Regardless, all of this is meant to stimulate your thinking and help you create a strategy that allows for you to gain the most out of your investment, not discourage you by any means. If you can think of these items while you move to and through product selection, you will be more alert to what you need to know and what will work (and not work) within your environment.

Last but not least, be alert and aware of overselling. These days, everything is sold with a large number of services you don't need or, worse, can't use, which increases the cost. Another type of overselling comes with modular systems. With modular systems, you can cheaply buy portions over time, but by the time you acquire the fully functional system, the cost is higher than buying the regular product. Both of these marketing plans are made to increase your expenditures but in two different ways. Be aware of them both, and as you move to product selection, research and ensure that what you get is what you need. There is a saying in the corporate finance world, "It's hard to go back to the well," which means that once upper management has allocated initial funds, they're unlikely to give you additional money later. Be aware of both of these marketing techniques when considering product vendor and offerings.

WARNING   Be careful when talking with vendors about their platforms and capabilities. Most times you will want to move into a solution at your speed and pace, not theirs. Also, you may need to consider that often the AIOps platforms a vendor may sell will only become fully functional (or realized) when you run their systems exclusively and simultaneously. So, mixing platforms (especially when considering open-source solutions) may not always work correctly or may require advanced configurations that increase the overhead on managing the system you are deploying.

AIOps Platforms, Products, and Services Selection

Product selection can be tricky. Since AIOps is a newer technology offering that everyone seems to be interested in, it's hard to navigate the marketing and modular nature of the products offered today. Use the first part of this chapter to help you prepare to navigate these aspects of the strategy process by creating a goal statement, defining a basic scope, and understanding the basics of marketing, finance, and how project management plays a role in the AIOps platform deployment. In this section, I will explore some of the biggest and most widely used products in AIOps today. Among these are the Gartner Magic Quadrant top picks as well as others that healthcare systems use to achieve artificial intelligence operations management to reduce time to resolve, help prevent issues, or correct them through automation.

Once you navigate the "gotchas" and work through the tough questions, you will see the bright side of AIOps. In other words, yes, there is a light at the end of the tunnel. The light is a bright one that can bring your infrastructure and operations to the next level and ideally, over time, reduce IT incidents, and issues, and/or provide the ability to resolve issues more quickly and expediently. Production selection can be difficult, and my initial advice to you is to take your time and review your options carefully. There is no rush to get through the initial scoping and product selection. If you pick the wrong thing and pay for it, in time you will really "pay for it."

AIOps Product Selection: General Topics

Selecting the correct products can be difficult, but not impossible if you know what to look for. In this section, I will highlight three product offerings that we will reference throughout the book. They are industry leaders, have longevity in the market, and are in the Gartner Magic Quadrant. Before we begin going through the selected products, you should understand what the Gartner Magic Quadrant means to you when scoping your project. Gartner, Inc. (gartner.com), is a large information technology service management (ITSM) company that provides consulting, advising, documentation, and marketing assistance to those who work with them. It's a well-known company that many in our industry have used at some point. It is also reputable, with industry experts working within the ranks to provide not only best-of-class service, but the experience and knowledge to back it up. One of the services that Gartner offers is through their documentation and marketing section called the Magic Quadrant. The Magic Quadrant is used to help buyers understand where the market leaders sit in the specific space or specific function they claim to offer.

The Magic Quadrant carves up the competition into four quadrants where leaders, challengers, niche players, and visionaries can be plotted along two axes: completeness of vision and ability to execute. Gartner places organizations and products in quadrants based on the market data that Gartner collects, reviews, and then releases for consumption. For example, Dynatrace (`dynatrace.com`), a company we will review in our product selection, is a market leader in both the "completeness of vision" and "ability to execute" realms. The Magic Quadrant market research reports provide the specific information you may require to help refine your selection and scope the project based on your goal(s).

CAUTION   Gartner is just a company doing business. It is a great source of information and acts as a guide, but you should still research extensively when doing your analysis and workup of production selection. Nobody knows your organization better than those who work within it, lead it, and run it. Yes, there is always a need for help, and we do bring in experts and other consultants to lead the way. However, make no mistake, just like any other consulting firm, this company is looking to extend business beyond its initial consultation to include providing custom guidance to help with deploying of tools, services, and any other project deliverables.

Another important consideration when getting into product selection is what I like to call the "everything plus the kitchen sink" marketing mentality. Most companies want to corner the space and dominate the market. Therefore, they may already provide a feature-rich tool that may be missing a few bells and whistles that other companies can sell to you. Because of this, these companies sometimes purchase niche players in the market and then "bolt on" their tools to the broader portfolio package. Because of this, the companies' offerings may be disjointed and not work well together when they are newly merged. This is something to consider when looking at a product. These companies also want to sell you everything in a modular fashion, but you may not need or be able to use all of them at this time. That noted, many of these features can still be useful, depending on your circumstances.

Some of these features include the following:

- Application Performance Management (APM) is a series of tools used to measure and monitor the performance of applications used within your organization. For example, if you have an application in a healthcare system that provides medical records and want to know how this application is performing (baselining, usage, and metrics) against a threshold you set, APM will be useful.

- Cloud-centric systems have a cloud provider dashboard that offers usage, metrics, performance statistics, and other useful data.

- Digital business analytics and business intelligence (BI) systems provide other analytical offerings to include the review and analysis of critical data in your environment. For example, in healthcare you may want to better understand population health management (PHM) or pop-health. The analytics performed could help find chronic health conditions and better understand them.

- Information technology service intelligence (ITSI) is the function of managing, monitoring, and planning actions revolving around service offerings in your enterprise. A service may be to provide a service delivery function such as service desk where this "service" can be maintained through an application dashboard monitoring data and providing service intelligence actions.

- All of these are offered in a "dashboard" tool that may come with any of these tools, or they may be a separate modular part of the portfolio of offerings, and only through the dashboard can you pull metrics and create automation functions where end users can log in and pull their own data or reports as an example.

These are all potentially important considerations in your strategy of deploying AIOps. The big areas that AIOps seems to cover in this spectrum are root-cause analysis and creating actions through automation, orchestration, workflow management, and alerting. Much of this can be done through ingestion of data from sources (ideally all sources) that you want to manage, monitor, and maintain. The reason why I am tying all of these together is that as you research every one of these AIOps platforms, you will absolutely see and be offered all of the functions that I just reviewed. It is important to know what they are, what they do, if they are modular, and, most importantly, what you ultimately need to service your goals. So, for example, if providing data metrics on the usage of application hooks in your environment is part of the scope,

AIOps may only provide a portion of that complete picture where the entire dashboard view may require APM as well. Make sure you are able to unwind each offering so that you have a clearer picture of what you need when you review your products.

Product Review: AIOps Tool Splunk

Splunk (splunk.com) purchased the SignalFx startup for AIOps integration and made an already robust, mature, and outstanding product into a tool that can provide more insight and functionality through the creation of actions, automation, and self-healing. Splunk is by far one of the market leaders in AIOps and has been around for many years providing big data analysis services for companies.

One of the roles Splunk originally played years ago was to ingest and review networking data, logs, alerts, and other critical data to draw a picture of network health in your environment. The ingestion of server data later helped to create a more complete picture of what may have been a problem. A common example would be that a set of end users couldn't access a service such as a web application. By reviewing the data in Splunk, it would have been possible to see that servers were providing Domain Name System (DNS) errors and were likely causing the issue, whereas all of the network components interconnecting the application to its clients had no issues at all. Prior to using a system like Splunk, an organization would likely open a phone bridge up, get all of the teams (network, server, desktop, etc.) on, and start to have each group check their respective areas. This was timely and a waste of resources.

Fast-forward to a fully deployed, maintained, and monitored system like Splunk. Now the help desk agent receiving the call could query the system and see that there were issues in a specific area and try to get the respective team online to fix it. If an issue requires further escalation and another group to review and resolve it, the entire process can be made faster and more efficient through the use of data from a tool like Splunk.

Splunk has grown into a mature company that helped start and revolutionize the movement of gathering and analyzing big data, and Splunk is now a market leader in this space. Their mantra is "turn data into doing," which they accomplish by using automation, orchestration, and AIOps to more effectively manage data.

Figure 3.2 shows Splunk providing a dashboard of all the data it receives in filtered modules that provide snapshots of health and integrity. In this figure, we can see Operational Intelligence, which is the end-state goal of a successful deployment.

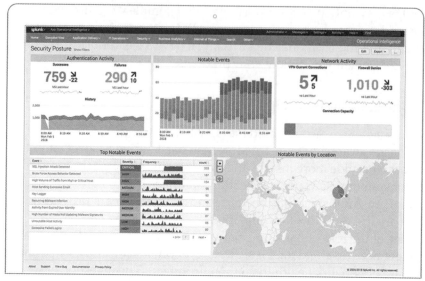

Figure 3.2: Viewing Operational Intelligence

In Figure 3.2, the deployment of Splunk reports that when filtering on security events, there are numerous issues that need to be reviewed and acted on. It may be that you build the automation directly into the system through AIOps so that when there is an issue (like a malware outbreak), your network access control (NAC) platform can take action and quarantine the systems spreading the issue. The dashboard can also be used so that you can configure alerts to go out as well as auto-mate the launching of a communication alert that gives key users an update on when certain thresholds are triggered or specific security events take place.

To deploy Splunk, I would recommend using the trial versions to get an idea of what you can use with the tools and/or engage their sales and marketing team to have a business manager and sales engineer walk through the tools and provide a demo. In Chapter 4, I will go through the specifics and details of deployment based on a project plan and its associated tasks.

Figure 3.3 shows the Executive View of the Operational Intelligence dashboard. The Executive View can provide a high-level oversight into how your organizational health looks and its current status. In this example, you can look at transactional data, latency of application usage, and the cause of the issue that is resulting in the alert. In Figure 3.4, you can drill down into each module to learn more about the health of your system and how it is operating. This ability to view in detail what the system is reporting is fundamental to AIOps with Splunk.

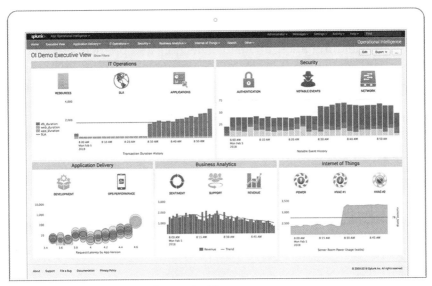

Figure 3.3: Splunk Dashboard Executive View

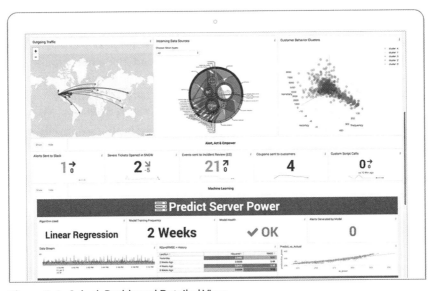

Figure 3.4: Splunk Dashboard Detailed View

This deployment becomes the groundwork needed to make AIOps come to life. Now that you have completely deployed the Splunk architecture into your environment, you can see that you have event management, correlation, alerting, thresholds, and dashboard monitoring established. To get the full benefit of AIOps, you need to configure actions based on root-cause determination, anomaly detection, and predictive analytics. This means you will need information technology service intelligence (ITSI) and a service analyzer to allow for root-cause management. You also need to set actions in the dashboard and establish configuration items (CIs) so that you can automate behaviors.

TIP   If you are looking to use Splunk (or any product reviewed here, you will need to look at how the company offers the deployment of its service, whether on-site or cloud-based. Most vendors provide their products as a service that you can subscribe to, which is often referred to as *software as a service* (SaaS) or *AI as a service* (AIaaS), both of which are discussed later in this chapter.

NOTE   Although you can get Splunk hosted, you can run most of the software, services, and systems in your environment, which makes it especially interesting to those who have an issue with taking their operations into the cloud. ServiceNow and Dynatrace both primarily exist in the cloud and in healthcare. There is a challenge with getting executive leadership to agree with moving operations outside their walls to the cloud. This is not because they are trying to cling to their current system or refuse change, but more so to be cautious about what they perceive to be added risk. Healthcare information is sacred and needs to be protected at all costs. Putting this data into the hands of others has caused hesitation for most healthcare providers and systems to move into the cloud at full speed.

Product Review: AIOps Tool ServiceNow

The next market leader in the AIOps space is ServiceNow (service-now.com). ServiceNow has become the de facto leader in the IT service management (ITSM) space and is a Gartner Magic Quadrant leader. AI for IT operations management (ITOM) is the method in which ServiceNow promotes and markets their AIOps platform. Before I get too deep into ITOM and what it does, let's take a quick look at the actual ServiceNow offering and its modular approach to providing a one-stop shop for all service management within your organization.

One aspect to keep in mind when looking at a platform like Service-Now is that it's extremely expensive. The "everything plus the kitchen sink" marketing mentality of ServiceNow is that if you deploy it as your basic service desk system, it will provide you with the basic foundation for all other modular platforms like ITOM. For example, in Figure 3.5, you can view the event monitoring function within ServiceNow that can help to create actions based on issues in your environment. The theory here is, if you have ServiceNow deployed as a service desk system, the event correlation and alert will correspond to an action and create an incident ticket based on the corresponding CIs.

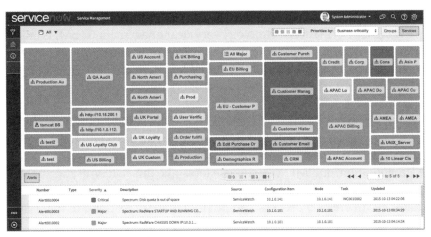

Figure 3.5: ServiceNow service management

Event management, correlation, and ultimately automation of the event will depend on how much of the system you have deployed and how complete the deployment is. This is loosely translated to a building block approach where you configure all systems in your enterprise in a configuration management database (CMDB) as configuration items that map to services. An example of one benefit of this is if a server hosting an application is not performing well, it will show up on the event management map as a dashboard item having an issue. At that point, the AI portion of the action will cut a ticket based on the appropriate CI violating threshold. Other actions can be configured, but the simplicity of just cutting a help-desk incident ticket based on the violation of a threshold is the rudimentary design of AIOps at its most fundamental level.

This should also demonstrate the importance of using your product selection and pilot time as a strategy planner, goal designer, and scope definer. If you do not provide the building blocks needed for the entire system to work, you will not be able to realize the AI or ML portion of it through the more advanced features of ITOM.

In layman's terms, ITOM is a fancy name for a heightened sense of alerting (and action creation) based on IT operations, which is really based on incident triage and response. All systems and services functioning in an environment are prone to issues, whether by failure of the system or service or by change through documented and undocumented change management. When properly configured, ITOM can help monitor and display data, automate events and actions to speed up root-cause analysis (RCA), help automate corrective action (CA), and reduce resolution time.

Much of information technology service management (ITSM) is based on service management fundamentals that can be traced to the Information Technology Infrastructure Library (ITIL). ITIL includes service design, service strategy, service transition, and operations and continuous service improvement (CSI). In the modular dashboard system of ServiceNow, Figure 3.6 highlights the use of CSI on key metric review through the Insights Explorer, which can be used to further create more helpful automated actions. So, for example, if you want to improve service through AI, automation, and ML, you can use tools like this to identify where you have impacts, performance issues, outages, events, and other alerts so that you can create a process and put it in place to respond to that issue.

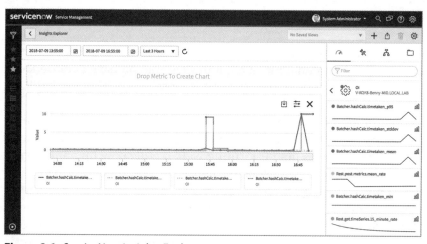

Figure 3.6: ServiceNow Insights Explorer

AI Insights Explorer is also self-service based (like much of Service-Now), which means that if you want to build your own dashboard with metrics to identify where you have issues, you can do so to work through problems. ServiceNow ITOM uses AI to better your IT operations through the main components of discovery, event management, operational intelligence, orchestration, service mapping, and cloud management if you are operating in or with a hybrid cloud provider.

The main design component that needs to be considered is the building block approach, where ServiceNow as a basic service needs to be deployed for ITOM to work with. When you add the ITOM component, you gain the other functionality that allows for self-healing. As an example, you can deploy and map a service in ServiceNow so that when an issue occurs, a ticket is cut as part of the incident management component where the issue is triaged, a priority is set, and you can view all affected components of that service.

If you have a hospital where clinical operations have been affected by an impacted service of the EMR, you will see that within ServiceNow. However, it will allow you to drill down and identify that the service may be affected due to an issue in the Citrix architecture that is causing your clinicians to not be able to pull up and use the EMR. ServiceNow will have a knowledge base that will likely be filled with information about what to do with an issue like this, or if you have AIOps components configured, you may have the service mapped to act upon the issue with an action. This means that if, for example, there is an outage of the EMR due to a problem with a Citrix server, the action may be to immediately move end users to a known good server in the server pool (likely filled with other Citrix servers) that can service the clients looking to use the EMR. This is where robust operational management is realized in the investment of self-healing. Note, however, that you need to configure these items and actions, and you have to rely on collected data, correctly configured CI information, a working CMDB, and ultimately, the resilience of the server pool redundancy for this example to be a reality when an issue takes place.

This is but one of many possible situations that can arise; however, it is a common one. It may be something you want to discuss with your vendor when scoping your project. Knowing and cataloging your top issues is important when developing your goal statement along with your initial project scoping exercise. Not knowing the problems you will face will hamper your ability to design the appropriate tools to handle them. If you can't design your tools to properly handle your problems, your tools can't provide all the benefits of ROI on reporting, take effective action on issues, and ultimately perform self-healing.

ServiceNow ITOM can also handle more than just orchestration and automation functions. It can help to provide metrics and insights into whatever service delivery issues you have so that you know where to focus your time when developing automation processes. The ITOM dashboard can help to show these metrics and insights and assist with developing predictive analytics, machine learning strategies, and AIOps solutions. The major module within ITOM event management that allows for ML, AI, and other automation functionality is based on operational intelligence that includes the ability to map the detection of issues to actions and prevent or self-heal them.

> **NOTE**   Take note that most if not all of ServiceNow's offerings are cloud based. Because of this, you may want to ensure that using cloud services is acceptable in your organization and that you have permission to do so.

Product Review: AIOps Tool Dynatrace

Dynatrace is a leader in the AIOps, APM, and other service management space. Similar to Splunk, ServiceNow, and ITOM, Dynatrace is a cloud-based SaaS provider. AI in a SaaS platform is sometimes called AI as a service.

One of the selling points for Dynatrace is that it is similar to Splunk, but not as overwhelming as ServiceNow. I tried to put three products on display here so that you, as the reader, can view different solutions that can be used to map to your goals. If you already have a service desk system and your goals are simply to automate service restoration and event management–based issues while hosting your systems in the cloud, then Dynatrace is your solution. Figure 3.7 shows the Dynatrace dashboard for managing and monitoring your cloud instance.

Davis is the name of the Dynatrace engine that provides AI functionality. Once you have your instance loaded and ready, you can start to populate it with the data needed to manage your operations. So, as noted earlier, you will have some discovery to do to get your systems loaded into the instance. Much like Splunk and ServiceNow, you can use predetermined data from a source such as a CMDB, or many of the applications available use a small agent deployed on the systems you want to manage/monitor and ingest into the platform, or in some instances connect directly to them via an application programming interface (API) or using Windows Management Instrumentation (WMI). The engine, Davis, is able to provide the AI function by scanning all data it has ingested during event management engagement and does so in real time. If your systems are not all in the instance and the engine does not have a complete picture of your enterprise, you will not be able to get the most out of the root-cause analysis, deterministic behavior, and self-healing processes of Davis, so make sure you apply this as part of your deployment strategy. It may also be difficult to do so with a cloud provider. That's why you need to also include the SaaS solution specifics as part of your design scope. Figure 3.8 looks at the data collected in real time and provides a dashboard view of events, correlation, and what your operations management looks like from a health check perspective.

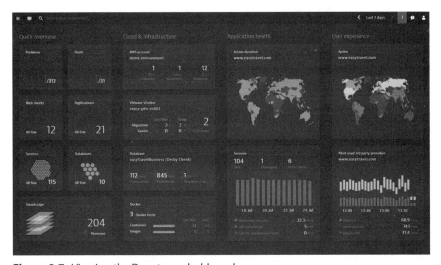

Figure 3.7: Viewing the Dynatrace dashboard

Another benefit to using Dynatrace is that it scrutinizes the data through continuous autodiscovery of any changes in your environment. As long as you have a complete mapping of your services and systems loaded within the tool, it can look for any changes to the environment and either alert on them or self-heal where appropriate. It can do this through the use of agents or APIs to and from your configured systems. As shown in Figure 3.9, this dynamic view of change can be monitored from a dashboard that allows you to see how everything is connected in your environment and, more importantly, how it cascades services (service mapping) so that if something is impacted (or an event is triggered), you are able to determine how that may further impact service delivery.

This section explored some aspects of how to map a strategy prior to purchase. The key here is to know what you want to get before you get it so that you don't waste time, money, or any other resources that can impact you and your organization.

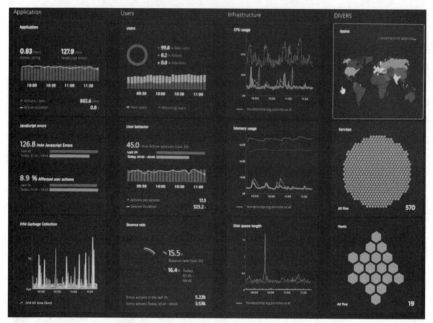

Figure 3.8: Drilling into the data with Dynatrace

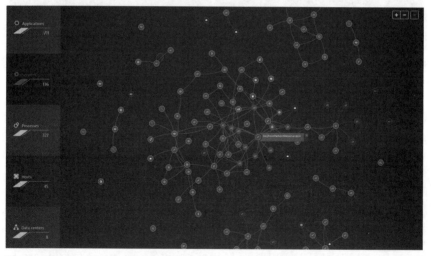

Figure 3.9: Service mapping dashboard

Workflow and Event Management Design

In this section, I will discuss other factors that are important when considering the strategy and design of putting an AIOps platform into your environment. So far, I have discussed the need for a service desk function to triage incidents and create a ticket as part of the automation of AIOps. I have also mentioned a need for an appropriate tagging of assets in your environment as CIs. This also translates into the population of a single source of truth (SSOT), which may be your CMDB. Change functions are key because you will want to manage any unexpected or unwanted changes in your organization's operation. There are also changes generated by growth, expansion, mergers, application upgrades, and migrations. There is a lot to consider, but this chapter and Chapter 4 should provide a great foundation for identifying and procuring an AIOps system that is appropriate for your enterprise.

Service Design with AIOps

When deploying AIOps in your enterprise, you will need to also consider other key components used in many large-scale enterprise infrastructures besides what you want to monitor. One of the most foundational elements is your company's service desk or help-desk system. This is usually the place where most of the incident management, incident triage, prioritization, and process handling occur. Because your AIOps platform will automate much of the work that needs to be done, it will have to cooperate with your service desk to handle tickets.

ServiceNow is in fact a service desk system with modules such as ITOM that handle AIOps and operations management functions. These two are part of the same unit, whereas Splunk is a system that will need to work with your service desk system to realize those benefits.

Designing the triage of events is the starting point for handling the workflows needed for automation, orchestration, and self-healing. Figure 3.10 shows how all your systems interact with each other, which is important because it affects how they will handle any outages or other issues at a server farm.

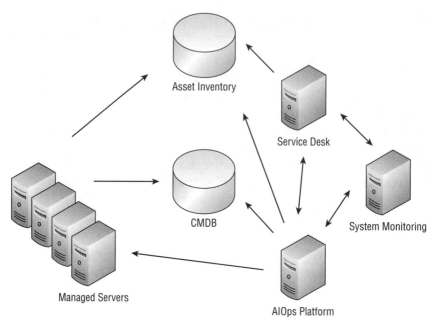

Figure 3.10: Service design with AIOps

How you design the triage of events will be based on how everything is configured to provide alerts. Here is a list of what is most common based on the example in Figure 3.10:

- An issue with the managed servers is detected by the AIOps platform, or an alert is captured by the systems monitoring tool of the servers, which then reports the issue to the service desk system or directly to the AIOps platform. The AIOps platform can also be configured to receive the same alerts from the servers themselves from an agent or API.

- The AIOps platform may attempt to self-heal the issue, regardless of whether the service desk system cuts a ticket so that the issue is documented and can be handled and escalated if needed. All of these items are kept as CI information in the CMDB or IT asset management (ITAM) system so that there is an inventory of the systems and what they do. They may be kept as service mappings in the service desk system.

- If the managed servers experience an issue such as a hard drive failure that causes the system to go offline, impacts service, and cannot self-heal, the ticket is raised in priority and brought to an engineer who will work to handle the issue.

■ If the AIOps system is able to self-heal the service, for example, it can move the service to an appropriate redundant node that may be in a cluster, the service may continue to function. In this case, the service has self-healed, not the system. The ticket will need to be updated so that a new drive can be put into the down node for it to be brought back online to serve as the backup if the production node goes offline.

We just explored a lot, and believe it or not, there is still more to consider. The goal of this book (and primarily this chapter's focus) is to get you thinking about these possibilities and the depth and complexity of what goes into the design and deployment of an AIOps platform appropriate to your organization that actually delivers on what it says it will by providing a return on investment (ROI). It will do this when these considerations are taken into the design process and laid out correctly to handle use cases like this one. If you find that your goal statement maps to common use cases, then this may be how you want to map your services and, more importantly, the actual self-healing functions that will allow for all of your systems to work correctly together during event handling, fault management, or other fault, configuration, application, performance, and security (FCAPS) management scenarios. Workflows and processes that appropriately handle anomaly detection and conduct actions are the goal. This is why tuning and postdeployment refinement are important. Common pitfalls to deployment (all or nothing) can be quickly identified by a use case like this one. If you're only capturing minimal data, how can you realize the benefits of AIOps? Or more specifically, if you don't have good data like CIs in a CMDB that is accurate and updated (for example, as systems are changed, maintained, ingested, and so on), how can an AIOps platform be accurate? These considerations must be reviewed prior to deployment.

Day-to-Day Operational Management

Your postdeployment picture should be one that is complete and has had a full ingestion of data, the data is maintained and updated, the AIOps platform of your choice is operating and able to identify issues, and, in most cases, it can self-heal issues, which is the epitome of success in this scenario. You will still need to maintain the system. Like any other IT system, constant care and feeding are required. AIOps has an interesting marketing concept: deploy AIOps to reduce your footprint. However, deploying/maintaining an AIOps platform increases your footprint. There is no escaping the fact that you will need to manage, monitor, maintain, upgrade, and continue to handle your service as well as the hardware it runs on. If in the cloud, the business liaison with the provider will need to be maintained as well as the financial and legal components. The true benefits of an AIOps platform are the speed of identifying issues, solving them through self-healing when it can, and determining the root cause by bringing together groups quickly with a clue as to what the problem is, helping to reduce the silos in organizations. These benefits do not always require a reduction in workforce. You're putting another system into your organization, and it needs to be managed by someone, which can often mean keeping your existing workforce and shifting their responsibilities.

The use case presented in Figure 3.10 shows other systems that need to be integrated with and monitored/managed as well. Service desk tied in with day-to-day management and operations is critical. As a leader in the organization, you will need to pull metrics and ensure that KPIs and CSFs are met, identify trends, and use this data to create ongoing and future strategy. Monitoring and general operational response to events, triggers, and alarms needs to continue. You will gain a lot of insight, and when self-healing responses are put in place, a reduction in workload will happen; however, tickets will be created and managed, and the AIOps platform may not always get it right. For example, in the use case I provided in Figure 3.10, the service was restored, but the problem was not fixed. It requires the ticket to be assigned to the appropriate party that can order, procure, and deploy the new hard drive to restore the system to 100% functionality. Healthcare clinical outcomes from AIOps can be made better, but make sure you are well versed in talking about what the true benefits are, as well as how long it may take to realize the benefits of self-healing, what is realistic, and what is not. Not all problems can be solved by AIOps, so make sure you know what problems it does solve and why.

Summary

Artificial intelligence in operational models has become the de facto standard of how services are designed and deployed. This is especially true in highly critical services such as those delivered by healthcare where lost time, mistakes, and administrative red tape impact the patient experience negatively. With more push toward "zero" downtime and less impact on 24/7/365 systems, having the "intelligence" to continuously deliver accurate results is one of the most exciting technological developments in our time. This book will help you learn about AI and its importance in healthcare and provide practical examples and advice on how to actually deploy it in your environment to achieve positive outcomes. In this chapter, I have addressed the specifics of devising a strategy that can be used to start the procurement of an AIOps platform for use in your organization. Some of these specifics included creating a goal statement, looking at use cases, defining a strategy to handle product selection, scoping the project so a product could be decided on, looking at which current product and vendors are market leaders, deciding what systems reside on premise and/or in the cloud, knowing how to handle the deployment of these systems, and looking at many of the caveats that may occur. Setting expectations, knowing what products provide, understanding their modularity with other services like service desk and APM, and recognizing how these systems all interconnect and interoperate are all critical when selecting a product for use.

In the next chapter, I will expand on what we learned in this chapter with a focus on the project phase, what needs to be done to deploy an AIOps system, and the importance of resource management and usage before, during, and after deploying the system.

Project Planning for AIOps

"Measure twice, cut once."
—Unknown

Now that you have taken the steps to prepare an AI operations (AIOps) deployment in your organization, selected a product, and conducted a proof of concept, you need to begin the planning phase of deployment. Once it's deployed, you can customize, build, develop, and automate workflows and other logic to bring value to your platform. As you strategize and deploy AI operations into your healthcare setting, the main focus will be doing so correctly, and that requires an understanding of what the project will look like and what project planning fundamentals are required.

This chapter discusses the requirements of building a project plan that you can use to deploy AIOps in your organization. In Chapter 3, I covered some of the basics of planning, but focused more on product selection and understanding the scope. In this chapter, we expand on the scope to help design the project plan, requirements, tasks needed to complete the work, resource assumption, and deployment phases all the way through installation and deployment of agents and ingesting data.

In the following sections, I will explore the requirements for deploying AIOps in your organization. All good deployments come from great planning and coordination. Luckily, project management allows for the use of a project manager (PM), tools, knowledge, and skills that allow for large-scale projects (such as the deployment of AIOps) to be broken down into manageable tasks that are backed by time, resources, and capital.

CAUTION   You may ask yourself if a project manager (PM) is really required to deploy AIOps into your organization. Your answer will be based on many factors you will learn about in this chapter. What is the size and complexity of the project? How many resources are you managing? Will it become too much while you work on and worry about your current responsibilities? These are questions you need to ask yourself early in the process of deploying an AIOps solution. My suggestion to you is to use a PM if you can. It will allow for a focused and dedicated approach to the project and help with the many groups you will need to work with during the deployment. Getting a PM will be really worth it if you can afford it.

Project Planning Requirements

The need for project management principles to be applied to your enterprise deployment cannot be emphasized enough. If you decide to build and manage the project yourself or work alongside a project manager as one of the stakeholders, using project management principles and solutions will really help with the success of your deployment. There are many project planning requirements, but I will break them down into manageable chunks as we move through the chapter. You can use the project planning methods that are presented as building blocks to get your project off the ground and shape out its scope. In Chapter 3, I discussed the scope refinement and product selection. This is not necessarily a pre-project requirement, however. I separated it because I wanted to show you how to identify needs versus wants and really frame what you need for your enterprise without worrying about or working through the actual rollout itself. The truth is, you can put the scoping, proof of concept (POC), prototype development, testing, and so on right into the first phase of your project plan. This is where we will start after you get through selecting a PM, developing a responsibilities chart, establishing a communications plan, and identifying resources needed to get the project started.

Assigning a Project Manager

The selection, hiring, or designation of a project manager is the most critical decision you can make. You could do the task yourself, but the deployment of AIOps into your organization is a large-scale effort that ties together the deployment of connectivity and/or agents to other systems, the management and monitoring of an enterprise-wide operations platform, the connection between many different groups within the organization, and the communication of this effort at all levels of the organization's staff and leadership. It is a big undertaking.

If you do decide to bring on a PM (or even do it yourself), there are a few things you should consider in the selection process.

- The PM should have experience deploying a large-scale, enterprise-wide application into an environment.

- The PM needs to have worked in a large environment, preferably one in healthcare so that there is someone who can connect the stakeholders, information technology experts, clinicians, and other staff during this deployment and keep them informed.

- The PM needs to have financial experience with contracts, licensing, and working with vendors (such as those we discussed in Chapter 3), and the ability to track resources inside and outside the environment.

The selected PM should possess this experience prior to selection. Obviously, if you can get an experienced PM, one who is certified as a Project Management Professional (PMP) and has Scrum, Lean, Agile, and other types of experience, you will fare even better in your deployment. Not all of these are going to necessarily guarantee a successful deployment, but having someone solely focused on and working with all of the different parts of the enterprise while deploying this intricate application will serve you well in the end.

TIP   Another important concept to consider is the product lifecycle. Many times, PMs will deploy a project and say it's completed when the tasks are done and the system or services are deployed. With AIOps, there is a need to make sure we manage the effort beyond the project lifecycle and through the entire product lifecycle, which means continuing to manage it. This will help you create a successful deployment because there will be a lot of post-project deployment tasks that need to be managed and maintained, such as tuning the system, updates, upgrades, and more.

The Agile methodology is a common framework in project development that allows you to flexibly adapt your approach as you proceed. Scrum is an Agile framework that breaks down the project deployment process into a series of manageable units called *sprints*. Figure 4.1 shows the layout of a simplified overview of how Scrum sprints work. A sprint planner is responsible for overseeing each sprint and its review. The sprint planner coordinates with the project team, which meets in daily meetings to discuss the progress of the current sprint. Your PM would likely either serve as the sprint planner or delegate that role to someone on the team.

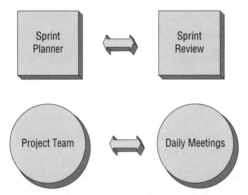

Figure 4.1: The Scrum framework's sprints

Scrum.org is a great reference (and toolset) for generating and using sprints. The framework it provides is simple and takes a lot of the lengthy work a normal project would entail and cuts it down into tasks that run down lanes and work in parallel. Depending on your project dependencies, you can get multiple work streams done in tandem, communicate as a project team (or group) as they occur, and work through them.

Another benefit to the Scrum framework is that when issues occur, you can use immediate team collaboration to solve problems, which works great for complex product sets like AIOps. You may have multiple teams working together to deploy the system and handle project resource contention, as well as any setbacks that create project scope creep. Figure 4.1 shows that the project team through daily meetings (sometimes called *huddles*) takes tasks, sets them as sprints (reviewed daily), and plans (or handles) them. This is just one example of how you can manage your complex project with more efficiency.

Creating a Project Plan

Once you have a scope, have identified the platform you would like to use, have a PM in mind, and have procured the AIOps platform of your choice, you will need to deploy. There is no better way to manage that deployment than with a project plan. A project plan is quite simply a set of tasks outlined in groups (normally called *phases*) that allows you to identify what you need to accomplish and when.

These phases of tasks can be developed further with resources assigned to them so that dependencies can also be mapped out. This becomes what is called the *critical path*. Once all of this is mapped out in Microsoft Project, Excel, or whatever project planning application or template you choose, you can see how things impact each other based on resource requirements and sometimes constraints.

At this point, you have the fundamentals of a project plan in your possession. I have kept this discussion of project planning relatively simple and at an overview level to make it more accessible for the reader. Entire books on project planning are available if you want to explore the topic in more depth.

> **NOTE**   You can certainly deploy AIOps in your environment without a project plan; however, the use of one will certainly provide a greater level of management of the tasks and a more streamlined approach to deployment and help you manage the myriad of tasks and resources required to successfully deploy it.

Your next step would be to map your plan to an assigned and sanctioned project with or without a project management office (PMO) within your organization. You may not have one and that is okay. In that case, you may want to work with your senior leadership (ideally most of them are stakeholders in the project) to help communicate the needs of the project and the changes it will bring. This can also be managed by the PM who should have a communications plan as part of the overall project plan to have weekly (or other specified time) meetings to keep all parties updated on the project status. From there, you can simply develop the project plan, manage it, and ensure that everyone stays in the loop during the project lifecycle as well as the product lifecycle.

Building the Project Plan

When building a project plan for AIOps, it is important to keep in mind that every project is unique and each project plan can look different. There is not a one-size-fits-all solution, and depending on the scope and complexity of the project itself and the organization it will service, there can be a lot of differences. In this section, we are going to deal with AIOps deployment situations in healthcare environments that are likely to be similar to what you have encountered in your field. I will share my experience with you and discuss what has been done in real-world situations and what turned out to benefit the organizations and leaders who adopted these concepts.

Figure 4.2 shows a sample project plan laid out in Microsoft Project 2020, or simply put, Project. Project is one of the leading programs used today to create and deploy project plans, although there are others.

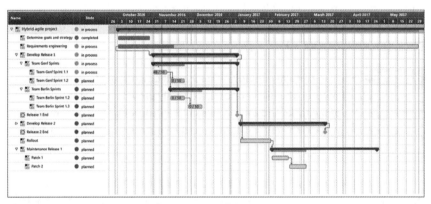

Figure 4.2: A sample project plan in Microsoft Project

> **TIP**   A deeper project management concept to consider is the use of a
> program or program management. The project we are creating may be a
> subproject in a bigger program in your environment. If that is the case, a
> project manager (and program manager) is required to help you manage the
> interconnectivity between projects that may impact each other. For example,
> dependencies across projects, resources assigned to many projects, and so
> on, can be managed at a higher level with program management. Just be
> aware of this since large-scale healthcare systems usually have a PMO and
> follow guidelines for programs as well as projects. Also be aware that this
> may all fall under a portfolio of programs and projects and be managed at an

even higher level. Since AIOps is a large product that touches across projects, you may have to consider this when you strategize its deployment within your organization.

There are a variety of ways to manage your project other than using Microsoft Project. Project planning based on the Project Management Body of Knowledge (PMBOK) or using sprints can be done by using either a tool such as Microsoft Teams or the Agile approach. It doesn't matter which tool or approach you choose as each will help you organize and deploy your project. However, each one uses different methodologies and layouts that help to streamline the use of multiple resources, the deployment of information and communication, the ability to get real-time responses from those working on tasks directly, and so on.

Stakeholders are the key to your project plan, project management, and product lifecycle's success. Financial resources (as well as human resources) are normally tracked and allocated. Therefore, having the right people behind the project and looking to make sure it is successful is going to play a large part in the product deployment and successful rollout.

ROI AND YOUR PROJECT PLAN

Understanding costs is crucial in an AIOps environment. Expectations and a timetable for return on investment (ROI) must be fully discussed and established with stakeholders. Similarly, stakeholders should be made aware that AIOps is a tool that once deployed needs time to be tuned, learned, further deployed, and then over time configured to take actions such as self-healing.

The project plan may have several phases. At the last phase of the project (which may take months to get to), you might find that your systems need to be fully configured with agents. You might also find that for your project to work with the AIOps system, after configuration is complete and data collection takes place, further configuration may be necessary and actions taken based on that data. A simplified example would be that you want the network to self-heal based on an outage. Similarly, if a circuit is degraded, you might want another one to be used.

Some of these things may require advanced configuration after the AIOps platform has been operational for some period of time. Although you might be able to project possible ROI in advance and track some limited ROI during early configuration and operation, true ROI may not be fully quantifiable until your AIOps platform has had time to establish its full benefits. Make sure you manage the stakeholders' expectations carefully, especially when discussing ROI.

The human resources for your project are also critical. When you build your tasks out in the project plan, you also need to fill out the resource sheet so that you can allocate resources to tasks. This not only allows those assigned the tasks to help manage their time and efforts, but holistically it helps the PM manage the project along the critical path and through any issues, resources challenges, dependency problems, and so on. Those selected for the project should be not only skilled at what they do but also knowledgeable of AIOps, especially in a healthcare environment.

This brings up the topic of training. A large part of a deployment is bringing everyone up to speed on the project, the product, the benefits, and the outcomes. Having seen a great many projects both succeed and fail in my time, I can say that training (and disseminating knowledge about the project and product itself) is a great way to avoid failure. Sometimes, dedicating a portion of the budget is necessary to establish a sufficient level of training.

Those who are deploying AIOps into an environment may know very little about the technology. For example, they may be network, server, or application experts, but they do not have a background in information technology service management (ITSM), configuration management, asset management, enterprise monitoring, automation, and other skills that one would deem fundamental for deploying and operating an AIOps solution. You may get more out of your project deployment if you opt to set up training classes for those who need to get up to speed on this new technology.

Another major component of pre-deployment, post-deployment, and moving into the product lifecycle is the responsibility assignment matrix (RAM). Setting responsibilities up front avoids confusion through the entire process of deploying AIOps. For example, most RAMs are further developed into what is called a RACI *matrix*. RACI stands for responsible, accountable, consulted, and informed.

A RACI matrix, as shown in Figure 4.3, is normally laid out in a chart where you can see all the deliverables or activities required to manage a project and the team members who are responsible, accountable, consulted, or informed for each of them. A good example would be the owner who is responsible for the AIOps system and its ongoing health may be the enterprise tools monitoring team, but those who manage the actual systems on a day-to-day operational level (perhaps the operations center staff) may be accountable. The programmers who handle the automation tasks may be consulted for their expertise, and senior leadership may be consistently informed of updates and priorities.

ROLE — Project Deliverable (or Activity)	Project Leadership					Project Team Members					Project Sub-Teams					External Resources			
	Executive Sponsor	Project Sponsor	Steering Committee	Advisory Committee	Role #5	Project Manager	Tech Lead	Functional Lead	SME	Project Team Member	Developer	Administrative Support	Business Analyst	Role #4	Role #5	Consultant	PMO	Role #3	Role #4
Initiate Phase Activities																			
Request Review by PMO	A/C					R/A	A/C	C											
Submit Project Request		I				R													
Research Solution						R/A	A/C	C	C			C	C			C	A		
Develop Business Case		A/C	I	I		R/A	C	C	C			C	C			C	C		
Plan Phase Activities																			
Create Project Charter	C	I	I	I		R/A	C	C	C	C		C	C			C	C		
Create Schedule		I	I	I		R/A	C	C	C	C	C	C	C			C	I		
Create Additional Plans as Required		I	I			R/A				I	I	I	I			C	I		
Execute Phase Activities																			
Build Deliverables		C/I	C/I	C/I	C/I		R/A	R/A	R/A	R/A	R/A					A/C			
Create Status Report		C/I	I	C/I	C/I		R/A	R/A	R/A							C	I		
Control Phase Activities																			
Perform Change Management		C	C	C		R	A	A	A							C	I		
Close Phase Activities																			
Create Lessions Learned	C	C	C	C		R/A	C	C	C	C	C	C	C			C	I		
Create Project Closure Report		I	I	I		R/A	I	I	I	I	I	I	I			C	I		

Figure 4.3: A sample project RACI matrix

A RACI matrix is a simple tool used by many PMs and other leaders who want to make sure that the role of managing a tool (such as AIOps) is clearly mapped to identifiable owners.

Another aspect of a project plan that helps the project planning process is the communications plan. A communications plan is simply a series of meetings, calls, updates via email, or whatever else the PM decides (and is agreed to by the parties involved) so that constant communication about the project is maintained. For example, you may have a weekly call with the project resources team but a biweekly call with the stakeholders. All parties get the project updates and artifacts from both meetings monthly in a compiled update. Keeping everyone informed and keeping open communications are the lifeblood of any successful project.

Figure 4.4 shows a sample of an AIOps deployment project with a communications plan that brings all important stakeholders together for the benefit of moving the project forward successfully. Important considerations about this team include the following:

- Stakeholder relationship management is an important consideration for a PM. You need to know how to select stakeholders and/or work with those selected for you.

- Stakeholder analysis and engagement will help you to identify key stakeholders up front as well as how to work with them on an ongoing basis.

- Stakeholders are often executive leaders in the organization. Their time is limited, and if wasted, it is costly.

- As a PM, you need to know how to communicate with this team in real time as well as in planned meetings. Reviewing the methods of communication, as well as their timing and frequency, is important for successful planning.

- Being able to define stakeholders' concerns and issues while keeping the project on track is important. You need to understand each stakeholder's level of commitment and resistance as well as influence.

- You should ensure that all areas of importance are considered and communicated with stakeholders.

- Make sure you create and use a communications plan and maintain a continuous dialogue between all parties as needed. You should obtain their feedback, make sure they stay involved, and use executive leaders for approvals and other necessary decisions.

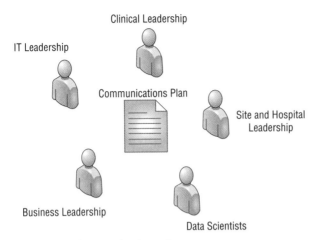

Figure 4.4: Communications plan

You can create a communications plan (also called a *stakeholder communications plan*) that can help you outline whom you need to contact and communicate with and at what intervals. Regardless of this, you need to also consider impromptu ad hoc meetings if you run into a project planning issue that can derail, change the scope of, or hamper the AIOps deployment in anyway.

Planning a Healthcare System Project

Now that I covered the basics of project planning with AIOps and its importance as well as the basics for getting a project off the ground, I would like to focus on the differences in the healthcare environment. There aren't many differences, but they are significant.

Healthcare is one of several fields that are considered essential to society. It is crucial to ensure that financial systems are operational when needed because their failure, even if only temporary, could cause chaos and widespread panic. The same is true for airlines, nuclear facilities, government, military, police, and many other critical facilities. However, the healthcare field is even more critical because innumerable lives are constantly on the line.

Beyond that, healthcare projects that go wrong can cause damage to your organization's reputation, which can result in distrust and fear in patients and their families. Imagine visiting your loved ones in a hospital, and the medical staff can't access the medical records to correctly distribute medication. This is why planning anything in healthcare needs to be done carefully.

Because of these concerns, when you deploy a system in a healthcare environment, there needs to be buy-in and approval of doing so at many levels. An example would be, if I were to suggest and propose the deployment of an AIOps platform, the health system would consider it and want to know the benefits of doing so. Since most of this was covered in Chapter 1, I will simply state that if the senior leadership of the health system agreed to moving forward with this effort, there would need to be an allocation of funds to do so. This allocation of funds would take money away from expanding new health system facilities, upgrading hospitals, getting new care equipment, and many other things that are needed to run a health system. It's not an easy sell, so they normally want to know what the ROI is on making such a lofty investment. Normally the sales pitch to senior leadership is based on the final stages of AIOps deployment, which include the automation of events, self-healing, and similar AI-based benefits. The challenge here is, there are many risks to this not turning out the way it was intended. If there is any hesitation to groups allowing access to these systems, if some teams decide that they will prioritize something else over the deployment of AIOps, or if access to key systems is not granted (common challenges), then the time frame of the deployment increases, the risk of not having the event handling and automation features not realized grows, and the pressure to deliver becomes overwhelming. Setting expectations up front and keeping all stakeholders updated through your communication plan is the best way forward for all parties involved.

CLINICAL STAKEHOLDERS

Bringing clinical leadership and site leadership in as stakeholders and keeping them updated will help not only to deliver on your project but to work with clinical staff when changes need to be made, updates need to be put into production systems, and clinical systems need to be configured within the AIOps system. Implementing these types of changes at a hospital generally also includes dealing with downtime procedures.

Downtime procedures are a big part of change management in any organization but are especially important in healthcare systems because of how they interact with standard operations procedures (SOPs). SOPs are required to have clinical staff continue operations when technology is either impaired (unscheduled downtime) or being maintained (scheduled downtime). Downtime procedures usually entail what to do when a system is impacted. In the case of an EMR, normal SOPs would show how clinical staff can switch to forms, paper, and other ways to manage healthcare reporting, documentation, and navigating through the use of clinical systems (labs and prescriptions, for example) without the use of their normal system. Once the system is back online, these notes are all transcribed and added back to the EMR so that all records can be updated and client/patient history can be complete within the health record.

Here are some things to consider in your project plan when working with clinical and site leaders:

■ Working with site leadership to ensure that impacted systems (for example, no access to the EMR) are communicated and planned with clinical staff to select an appropriate time to go to downtime procedures.

■ Making sure the downtime procedures have been incorporated into your budget (likely operating costs) to pay for the extra staff needed to move to paper and/or put the notes back into the EMR once the systems are back online and restored.

■ Making sure that all plans have been reviewed, are approved, and are understood by all clinical leaders so that in the case of contingency, disaster recovery, or any other form of business continuity planning (BCP), there is a well understood path as to how to revert to the original state of the systems or back up and restore them if needed.

Most large healthcare systems have a PMO, which makes it easier to manage. However, smaller hospitals and medical facilities, practices, and offices will not. They may be large enough for an enterprise AI project but may not have the logistics, resources, and head count needed. All this needs to be considered when selecting, approving, and managing an AIOps project.

Deploying AIOps

Planning and strategy are the keys to a successful AIOps deployment. For the rest of this chapter I will focus on how to move from project planning to project and service delivery. From here on we can work together as a team to identify what you will need to succeed in getting an AIOps platform ready to go in your organization. For this section, I will cover one of the leaders in the field, ServiceNow (SN), and how you can organize beyond the project plan to deploy this tool and get it up and running. As we continue through the book, we can look at the rest of what you would do after installation and basic configuration, but for now, let's get AIOps up and running in your organization.

Deploying AIOps into the Environment

There are many steps to getting AIOps installed and in use in your environment. The first two chapters of the book taught you about AI and AIOps, while Chapter 3 gave you the ability to scope out your project, select your product, and prepare your project to become a reality. So far, in this chapter I covered how to get your project going and why it's important to plan. Your next step is to select that product and get moving with the actual installation of the tool.

> **WARNING**   Whether you select an in-house solution or one that is hosted in the cloud, you will need to be able to manage and monitor the system so it can be leveraged by your internal IT staff as well as by others who may use the system to gain information and review data or dashboards. Regardless of whether you install the system internally or host it externally, the need to involve your infrastructure, network, and security teams becomes increasingly important.

The first consideration is whether you will host this system internally or externally. Figure 4.5 shows two types of deployments that are similar except for what is on-premise and off-premise. For example, Figure 4.5 shows an endpoint computer (end user, client) that needs to use a system that has to be managed via the AIOps system. Regardless of whether the system is cloud hosted or internally managed within the organization's datacenter, the experience should seem basically the same to the client.

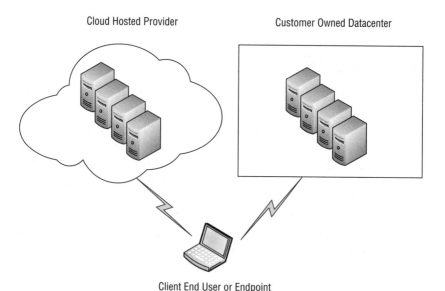

Client End User or Endpoint

Figure 4.5: Cloud-hosted versus internal solution

One of the reasons why the choice between internal local hosting and external cloud hosting is important is that you need to involve security, network, or other teams that deal directly with some of the differences. Sometimes the decision is already made for you, as in the deployment of ServiceNow. ServiceNow is hosted only on the cloud, and you cannot install an instance of it in your datacenter. When working with ServiceNow or another such cloud-hosted platform, you will likely need to ensure that connections to the cloud-hosted provider are appropriately sized (bandwidth, latency) and protected (encrypted). If you are using protected health information (PHI) or personally identifiable information (PII) in your systems, you will need to work with security to make sure that the data at rest and in transit is protected. There are many considerations that need to be made and more so when you connect to a third-party cloud provider.

The legal department may also need to be involved because contracts need to be approved, reviewed, and signed off on to use the instance on the cloud. There may be important legal bindings that require renegotiation so there are no issues moving forward or, if you need to back out of the instance, no issues getting your data back.

Deploying your healthcare AIOps platform will require you to consider all of the requirements up front, and this should take place in the first phase of your project plan. For example, if you want to deploy Splunk (in-house), you will need to know what servers or virtual machines it can run on, what the appropriate resources requirements are (disk, CPU, memory), where data is stored and kept (database), and all the other specifics of any IT deployment. This can all be found on the vendor's website, and you should make sure that you have reviewed it (or the appropriate teams have reviewed it) so that you know your deployment will be successful. You must also consider growth. For example, once you start to collect data, the size of disk needed (or database requirements) may grow exponentially and incur a sizable cost down the line; therefore, you may want to budget for this annually so that there are no issues moving forward when you need to grow your system.

Interconnecting systems is also a critical step to consider in the deployment of AIOps. So, if you are going to connect via an API or if you can use agents that collect data, all of that information needs to report back to the core servers. That means if you are traversing firewalls (cloud-hosted), you may need to add rules in a bidirectional fashion based on that traffic and its requirements. For ServiceNow, having the ability to connect to the instance over the Internet to the cloud-hosted provider will suffice. However, you need a contingency if your Internet links go down. Usually having redundant connections helps. Working with network services will allow you to design an appropriate solution where the right design will require redundant and resilient connections to the Internet, usually utilizing two different service providers and making sure that the points of presence and the central office (CO) are also diverse so that there is no way you will be totally out of business if you lose one connection.

One last consideration is if you do install these systems in-house and not on a cloud-hosted environment, you will avoid the monthly or yearly fees associated with hosting, which can be quite expensive. However, you will need to ensure that you have considered all of the costs of an in-house deployment in the same fashion you did with the cloud solution. Whereas in the cloud you do not have to pay for staff, server racks, electric bills, and the myriad of other IT and facility costs separately, you will still have to pay a bundled price that considers all of these items. When you deploy in-house, the same things are needed. However, those costs come directly to you and the organization itself. You are not in a situation of cost avoidance, but in a situation of making the management of it easier.

NOTE   AIOps platforms can also work together. In this chapter, I have mentioned ServiceNow and Splunk. ServiceNow works with the information technology service intelligence (ITSI) module of Splunk, and both can be used together. One of the benefits of using ServiceNow is that it is a true information technology service management (ITSM) tool and can adapt and incorporate the data from other trusted sources (like Splunk) to create tickets, correlate data, and use the data in event management and correlation for AIOps.

Configuring AIOps in the Environment

Once your scoping, project team, resources, budget, and stakeholders are in place and all parties are properly coordinated, you can then move to the actual procurement or deployment of the AIOps system. As mentioned earlier, there are a few ways this can be done. If you are cloud hosting, you will work with a deployment team and get your instance online and your systems connected to it for ingestion. If you are deploying in-house, your deployment team will install the systems, and you will prepare for the ingestion of data.

Self-learning will take place in time, once the data has been reviewed and trusted. Other learning mechanisms/methods will also be used so that automation can be configured and put into use. Service desk mapping will be one of the items you want to make sure is considered so you can appropriate triage and set escalation by ticket priority based on manual and dynamic alerts provided by fault and event management.

In Figure 4.6, you can see how the initial configuration may look with ServiceNow once you have all components online. For example, if you have a functional CMDB and trusted data sources configured correctly, you will be able to look at the event correlation dashboard and see how AI (and ML) take shape.

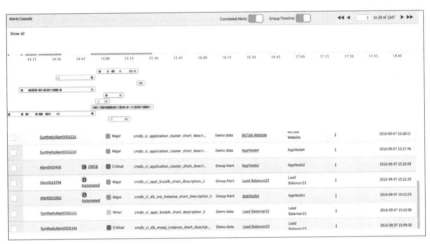

Figure 4.6: ServiceNow event correlation

Here in this example, we have alert correlation using machine learning (ML) to coordinate the first basic configuration of AIOps. For example, you can see the organization of alerts grouped together using temporal and stochastic relationships, which is the basis of time-series forecasting. This way alerts can be further correlated based on initial anomalies, the system reviewing how the alert binds to a service within the tool, alert actions, and root-cause analysis (RCA).

This is but a sample of what can be done. However, the keys are to have a fully functional CMDB and trusted sources of data configured into the system as well as all manageable systems ingested into the tool so that these relationships can be made. This is the basic building block of everything that we will learn in the next four chapters. If you do not have a fully deployed system, everything that we learn from here on to the end of the book will be flawed. How can you do true event correlation and automation or self-healing actions if only half of your network infrastructure is accounted for? How can this be done if only a quarter of your VMware servers are configured? This chapter underlines the basic need of you having all of the systems you want under the AIOps tool in the project scope so that you can manage all of it correctly without failure.

Once you have the initial configuration up and running, you can start to visualize how the rest of the system can be configured. For example, examine the layout I created in Figure 4.7. Here you can see a high-level, streamlined deployment of AIOps into your environment. When you deploy AIOps, consider this is a snapshot of a bigger deployment. For example, systems like VMware, Splunk, and Solarwinds (Solarwinds.com) interact with network events and systems events as well as systems configured in the CMDB. You can envision how they all are encompassed within the ServiceNow deployment (using ITOM for event correlation and AI automation and event handling) where tickets can be created and launched to operations teams that need to respond, while in tandem self-healing may be taking place in parallel for other issues.

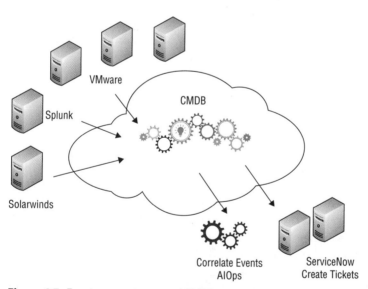

Figure 4.7: Event management and CMDB

As we close this section, remember it is important to create a strategy and plan a deployment correctly so that you get to this point where you can start to build on a strong foundation. The rest of AIOps is internal configuration and action generation as well as other types of configurations, but if you do not have the base system installed correctly and with good data, trusted sources of other data and a strong foundation, you will be hard pressed to move forward with a great deal of success. Do yourself a favor and give yourself the best chance at success by heeding the guidance provided not only in this book but in the vendor documentation also and the sales team you may be working with. Consider all of it and think through all case studies and possible scenarios. You need to have a good project team to deploy AIOps and do it correctly across your organization. You need to be in lockstep with the other teams to help realize this goal. Lastly, the leadership, stakeholders, and customers need to be just as involved as the rest of the team and communicated with frequently. By doing so, you can create good risk avoidance while moving the project through to completion.

Summary

Having a project plan in place is fundamental to deploying AIOps into your environment. Having a project manager, different types of project dependencies, a scope, a critical path, and resources are all important parts of project planning. Projects in a healthcare system share some similarities but also have differences compared to other types of projects. Lastly, the initial deployment and configuration of AIOps into your environment helps you prepare for the next section of the book where we will focus on the more advanced considerations that get AIOps to produce for you a system that allows for better event management, correlation of events, automation of actions, and efficiency in mean time to resolution (MTTR) as required.

Using AI for Metrics, Performance, and Reporting

"Excellence is never an accident. It is always the result of high intention, sincere effort, and intelligent execution; it represents the wise choice of many alternatives—choice, not chance, and determines your destiny."

—Aristotle

As you strategize and deploy AI operations (AIOps) into your healthcare setting, you will want to immediately reap the benefits and rewards. But you don't accomplish that by chance; it is the fruits of the choices made by deploying high-end tools to make an impact. What impact is made on the clinical side of the equation? Have you been able to reduce mean time to recovery (MTTR)? Have the automation and workflow enhancements made a significant impact on production? Have they reduced outages and relevant incidents? Has return on investment been achieved? All of these questions are asked prior to the deployment of AI, and the best way to find this information and prove that your answers are correct is within the tools themselves and the data you can mine from within. Specific tools, methods, and efforts can help to provide the data you need to get this accomplished. In this chapter, we will look at the tools and techniques you can use to achieve this goal.

This chapter discusses how to use AI and AIOps tools to identify service performance, looks at metrics for typical key performance indicators and critical success factors, and explains how to report on the outcomes of using AIOps to stakeholders, leadership, and those who have invested heavily in the products that have been deployed.

System Performance Metrics

After the system is deployed and ready for use, the next goal would be to provide data of either the performance or lack thereof. Various factors could change the impact of the tools' performance and the metrics you are producing. Before even considering those, it is important to first lay out what your metrics will be and how you will report on them so that you can make any necessary adjustments as you continue to use the AIOps tool. For example, you may have a metric configured to show the reduction of mean time to resolve (MTTR). This is an extremely common metric that is also labeled a *key performance indicator* (KPI) for many operations-based systems and tools.

Before we delve into what AIOps can provide, there is a need to fully understand information technology metrics, data gathering (mining and analysis), and how to report on what matters as well as what to do about your findings. To begin this exploration, the following sections will talk about the fundamentals of IT metrics and reporting based on outcomes, needs, and performance.

CAUTION   I will be using MTTR as a KPI and example for gathering metrics throughout this chapter. It is commonly used especially in the world of technology operations. It is particularly important in healthcare operations because systems that are unusable could result in the hospital and practices not being able to use systems, which disrupts clinical work. Although MTTR stands for *mean time to recovery*, it is often used interchangeably with *resolution*. Resolving a problem or recovering from it can sometimes be used synonymously. If the system is up, you have restored service, but in the world of ITIL service operations and problem management, that does not mean that the problem is completely solved. Also be aware that the *R* in MTTR can sometimes be confused with other metrics such as mean time to respond and mean time to repair. In this chapter, our focus will be mean time to resolution.

Information Technology Metrics

Information technology metrics matter. A tremendous amount of money and time go into technology, and you need to be cognizant of investments made and whether they are or were worth the time and capital. The best way to identify return on investment (ROI) is by looking at service performance by way of data metrics collected over a period of time in order to understand if the investment was worth it, and if not, what needs to be done to make it worth it. Remember, there are ongoing software, staffing, and other costs that keep an AIOps platform going strong, which means you want to show how it brings value.

There are two complications to using metrics to show value. You need to be sure that data is accurate and not skewed. You also need to show meaningful metrics that really speak to value. Looking deeper into these two issues, we can see that it takes a meaningful effort prior to deployment to ensure that you stay ahead of these challenges.

For example, accurate data means that you are measuring data that talks to the story of the metric. I use this concept all the time with the managers I train. I call it *storyboarding* the metric idea before you deploy it into action. In traditional film and comic making, this means you come up with the storyline and create a small sample of what that would look like before investing a tremendous amount of time, money, and resources into it. For example, in Figure 5.1, you can see an example of a metric concept that I would like to deploy and what it would look like prior to deploying it. This helps me to know what data I need to start to gather to tell the story through the data. In this example, I put together known data over a small sample period of time. My goal was to see whether there was a story to tell that would justify the time and effort to continue data mining. Here I could see trends such as faster time to resolution where it was followed by a higher trend with peaking, which caused substantial impact to the organization. Because of this, I believe there is a story here worth telling and have justified the full investment in putting together the metrics needed for leadership.

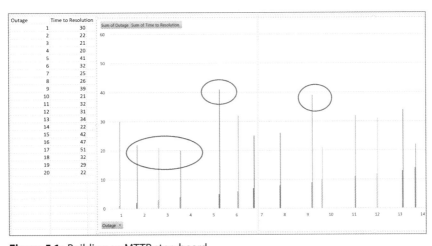

Figure 5.1: Building an MTTR storyboard

You prove the sample and then move forward with the full deployment. With AIOps, when we started to scope the project and come up with the deployment, the goal was to make sure that we encompassed all IT infrastructure so that the AIOps platform management of systems and ability to gather information, generate alerts, and strategize actions based on configured workflows would be complete and not missing large portions of important systems. In sum, this means if I only put network devices and desktop systems into the AIOps platform and do not look at the servers, I would not be able to accurately manage the enterprise nor would I be able to report on it accurately either.

To alleviate this problem, knowing what you want to report on as you strategize and scope the project would be the ideal situation to be in. For example, most commonly, MTTR would be able to be resolved only if you had a complete picture of all infrastructure in your AIOps platform, thus being able to report on it as being complete in the same manner. If you want to say you increased MTTR but you failed to include your Citrix servers that crashed once a week and did not register as an event in your AIOps system, your enterprise metrics would be skewed and not reliable to senior leadership who would be receiving them. The way to solve this would be to make sure that your metrics are covered by data that you pull reports from and on, and those data points would need to be reliable and complete.

IT metrics also need to be digestible by senior leadership. This comes in the form of reports and presentations that usually include graphs and other sources of data to help tell the story. Usually senior leaders want to know one thing: how does the investment provide value to the business? As you move higher up the ladder, the reports need to talk about providing value and how the money invested is being used in a positive way. Normally, many IT metrics provided by others can tell this story, but there will be times that leaders are left with virtually no understanding of what the value is, what the true impact on the business is, and, worse, how the money spent is an actual investment. It becomes tricky with AIOps because traditional operational platforms that provide fault management or other alerting functions can be easily reported on based on raw numbers collected from provided data points. For example, if we wanted to know how many times a server became unresponsive over three months, we can ask the system to generate that report and then dump that information into a table or chart to show a trend over time. It becomes more difficult when we say that when we want to use AI to proactively solve problems, how does that look on a chart? I explore those challenges and how to scale them in this chapter.

What you cannot rely on is the traditional metrics such as project completion dates but no information on the product lifecycle or its output of value. To say you deployed AIOps is the first checkbox to a completed system deployment, but it is by no means the last. In this section, I will lay out the most important pieces need to get meaningful reportable data from your AIOps system and how to show that it is bringing value.

RESEARCH FIRMS AND METRICS, PERFORMANCE, AND REPORTING

A great source of metrics, performance, and reporting information is Gartner and similar professional research firms. The data such organizations provide can be invaluable as you build your case to justify procuring large expenditures, increasing staff, and eventually achieving your desired return on your investments of AIOps.

Gartner and other professional research firms can provide a wealth of documents to help justify moving to AIOps, along with information on ITIL, metrics, service performance, reporting, executive-level reporting, and more. These organizations can provide help, support, or examples based on industry trends and use cases, such as the following:

- Examples of common metrics used in business settings
- Diagram examples of how metrics can be used to tell stories
- Reporting examples used in a series of different delivery mechanisms
- Best practices for all industries
- Use cases that fit your industry
- Current examples of AI, AIOps, ML, and other current technologies

When considering a serious approach to delivering executive-level reports that matter and make an impact, you can consider this chapter as a baseline on how to approach the topic, but if you seek more help, you should make use of Gartner and other professional research organizations.

THE IMPORTANCE OF ESTABLISHING BASELINE DATA

Before we get involved in the tools, planning, and strategy, there is a priority on understanding what a baseline is, why it's important, and how it relates to metrics and measurements. In all simplicity, baseline data is nothing more than a snapshot of data at a specific point in time. When I say *snapshot*, that can be an assessment, measurement, collection of state, or any other form or measurement such as threshold, size, frequency, rate, interval, and time.

An example would be if I wanted to establish a baseline of the amount of coffee I drink every day, I would record whatever that is over a month. If the answer is 3-4 cups a day every day for 30 days, then I have a basic baseline measurement. If I look at that rate over the next 90 days, I may see that it's closer to 3 cups a day every day for 90 days, and so on.

This is important because in the world of information technology and data science, if I wanted to spend money and forecast costs based on what I may need in a budget for the upcoming year, I would need to know what is currently in use but also what changes are taking place. For example, we may have been growing as a company and adding more servers each month. That means the bandwidth usage on my network may be increasing. So, if I took a snapshot of baseline data over 90 days and know that my normal bandwidth is about 10 megabits per second, if I suddenly added 250 more servers to the network, it's likely going to go up. By calculating this, I can make a mathematical prediction on how much more bandwidth I may need and increase it while I am adding the servers or prior to adding them.

This is why it is important to establish baselines as they are used as a comparison point for later deviations so that you can determine what planning you may need to do in order to deploy an AIOps platform. If you do the work and review the points made throughout the book on how to plan correctly, you can assess your own infrastructure and make these same mathematical predictions. In sum, you should consider the following areas as foundational items for taking baseline snapshots so you can plan your AIOps infrastructure correctly. Use the following as foundational items to review:

- Network bandwidth, usage, power, and capacity
- Server CPU, disk, and network usage
- Application growth and space requirements
- Storage growth and space requirements

Using AI for Metrics, Performance, and Reporting

Using AI for reporting, metrics, and performance can be challenging if you are unsure of what story you look to tell. As the previous section discussed, you can use the technique of storyboarding to determine what you would consider to be an acceptable breakdown of metrics, what your service performance is, and how to report it. Let's take a look at what each of these means:

- **Metrics:** You establish baseline data points (or markers) where you can identify trends, collect the data, and show it in a way that you can interpret using charts. Metrics can be derived from key performance indicators that are considered critical success factors (CSFs) used to tell the story of performance.

▪ **Performance:** System or service performance is what the outcome of the data collected and metrical representation tells us based on a specific amount of time, baselines set, and thresholds. For example, if you know that your MTTR is showing that if a ticket comes in it is resolved within 30 minutes or less and that is acceptable (and the norm), then that is your baseline or threshold. If you report on metrics for a specific period of time and it is showing that you are currently trending 40 minutes or less (10 minute differential), then that means something changed, and you should try to find out why this change has happened.

▪ **Reporting:** When you report, you take the metric data based on what your performance is or is not telling you and provide this information to leadership or other teams to either discuss what the results are or discuss what needs to be done next to fix any deficiencies.

Once you have an acceptable version of what a full report would look like, you can start to probe your system for the needed information to collect your data points. There is good news: almost all modernized system tools, programs, applications, and platforms generally have the ability to do metrics, measure performance, and generate reports directly from the tools themselves.

This does not negate that need to understand how to create the storyboard and understand what data points are needed and what your own organization's recognized and accepted service performance thresholds are. I have seen many times the reporting of misunderstood data or, worse, data that does not truly represent what is indicated by the report being given. For example, if we pull a report from the tool and see that MTTR is in acceptable limits but the operational teams are reporting that it is not, there is a clear misrepresentation. This is why it is imperative to know how to construct these factors outside the tool and then use the tool to create what you need based on your understanding of said factors.

Using AI to generate data for metrics, service performance, and reporting can be extremely helpful to prove out and promote ROI. When you have a fully functioning system where all of your infrastructure is encapsulated into the system and you have collected data for a period of time that can show a trend (positive or negative), you can get a lot of great information from the tools. In the coming sections, I will show you how to generate that information and show it to tell the story you need to tell. To see the entire process and how a workflow may appear, in Figure 5.2 we can see an AIOps platform in use with service performance data being sent to or being collected from data points set within the system. For example, the system may be sending data such as number of alerts generated per hour. This is derived and processed into a usable set of metrics. (This may be set to industry-standard KPIs.) You would then be able to generate and use a report or report to leadership on your finding. Later in the "Helpful Tools You Can Use" section, I will show you tools that you can procure to generate that information from the system itself.

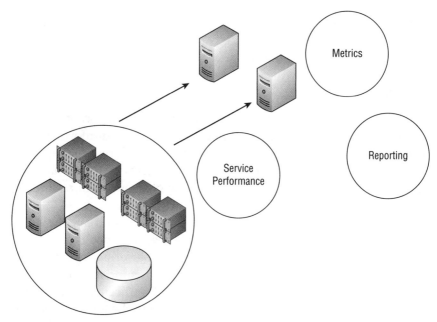

Figure 5.2: AIOps data collection

> **NOTE**   Storytelling is the beginning of your path to reporting. If you can
> talk to the data and the storyboard, you can talk to your goals of reporting
> metrics and what leaders need to know. As with traditional storytelling,
> you should have a plot as well as supporting data to talk to your goal of the
> story. You can find more information by searching online to see how story-
> telling with data can help support your case when discussing information and
> reporting to senior leaders.

Strategy and Goals for AI Deployment

The goal of your AIOps deployment is to produce a return on investment. When you deploy a system that handles the majority of your operational needs such as event and fault management, ticket generation, alerting, and other functions, you are able to fundamentally review system performance, gather metrics, and produce reporting based on the systems' collection of information and data. With the correct data points, you can pull and create metrics and reports, or with most systems, you can automatically generate the information from built-in dashboards.

So, where does AI fit in? Artificial intelligence (AI) and machine learning (ML) when fused with operational tools will allow you to build on what you already have with the ability to create workflows and automation based on system and service performance, rules, baselines, data collection, and specifically what rules apply as the system begins to learn what is normal baseline activity. For example, if I were to storyboard this, when using Splunk, I may have a normal baseline of faults generated by wide area network (WAN) ports bouncing or "flapping" and creating event tickets. With a serious event, the network may remain or appear to remain stable, but performance will be degraded during the event. We may never see it as an outage, but it may appear in the tools and system monitors as an event nonetheless.

Without AI, the normal process would be to tune the system in a way that when this specific event took place, instead of cutting a ticket on every up/down event that takes place (could be thousands) and flood the help-desk system with data, we could set the system (or tune it) to reflect that this type of event (a flap) may require a parent ticket only and a text to a systems administrator to investigate. With an AI or ML solution, we could automate this to happen based on a rule we place in the system, or, if the system truly learned the event correctly, it would automate this process on the first flap as a nonevent and cut a ticket for processing.

In Figure 5.3, you can see the two paths in action. The first path would be the event (or fault) taking place and the AIOps system collecting and analyzing the data, acting on a rule that may be manual or automatic and then paging for help. In the second instance, if AI/ML were in use, the rule would simply "fix" the problem based on a programmed or automated function. In the next chapter, I will get into automation in detail, but for now it's important to understand how the system will react to an event based on what the system either is programmed to do or has learned needs to be done.

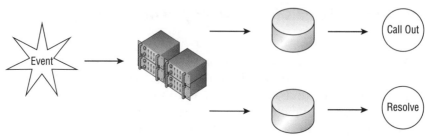

Figure 5.3: AI event process handling

Benefits of Healthcare AIOps Service Performance Reporting

The benefits of using AIOps to help support your healthcare operation cannot be understated. First, when measuring IT's business value, your journey with AIOps will be a marathon, not a sprint. Immediate positive impact comes from the ability to handle event management in a way where your teams are aware of any issues within the environment that need to be addressed. With a large platform like AIOps, the automation, workflow development, and advanced handling of issues come over time where the system can begin its learning process and make smart decisions based on analyzed data. This is where the marathon takes place. It is also noted by those with expert-level knowledge of these systems that this can be seen as a deployment of incremental developments, improvements, changes, and investments that once deployed and in use can help to deliver on realistic goals. Good outcomes and bad outcomes are both possible.

Let's first start with and quickly review the bad outcomes. Poor planning and unrealistic expectations result in bad outcomes. An incomplete deployment can result in a bad outcome. Not doing your research and strategy planning (as discussed in Chapters 1 through 4) may result in a bad outcome. Getting the wrong product for the job or your environment may wind up producing negative results and, thus, a bad outcome. Spending millions of dollars on a platform that is half-installed and not producing the results you need and therefore not producing return on investment is considered a bad outcome. The good news? The opposite of all of these negatives will produce the good outcomes I have strategized since Chapter 1. The reason strategy, scoping, and project planning are so critical to a successful deployment is that if you plan it out correctly, you can gain the insights you need and report them to leadership.

Outcomes based on performance data are critical to overall healthcare and health system planning. It is recommended you conduct the assessments to identify what your team is responding to, what systems suffer downtime, and what that impact looks like financially or just in resource time. For example, if you wanted to know that your critical systems and applications downtime has been low and uptime has increased significantly from your deployment of AIOps tools, you can then focus on other things in your environment instead of responding to outages. The benefits of artificial intelligence (AI) come from the reduced overhead of complex IT management of systems that requires significant time, resources, capital, and manpower. The other goal of being able to create good outcomes based on performance data is that you can provide your clinical partners with SLAs that really matter. For example, if I provide a service level agreement target of having system uptime at 4 nines (99.99 uptime), that means that I am on target with few downtime requirements that may need to put clinical systems, workflow, and those who manage the daily hospital and practice operations on alert when an issue arises. Downtime procedures cost health systems money. There is also a backfilling of data that needs to take place once all systems are online. Verification of data needs to take place. Good outcomes come from the clinical staff being focused on clinical work, not worrying about calling into a help desk or trying to resolve technology issues while providing clinical support. The following are the positive outcomes that can come from AIOps when deployment is a success:

- Saving money
- Empowering operators
- Automatically provisioning requirements
- Delivering value faster
- Capturing knowledge
- Documenting process and workflow digitally
- Having anyone be able to execute (ease of use)
- Less reliance on experts
- Reducing risk
- Orchestrating change
- Reducing credential access
- Standardizing executions

- Speeding process
- Directing requests from service catalog
- Creating new items quickly

Using AIOps correctly not only will be able to reduce the amount of downtime impact but can produce quality metrics that allow you to report on and show benefits of the tools you have invested in. This list is but a segment of top "wins" from deploying the tool correctly and completely.

> **CAUTION**   You should always try to underpromise and overdeliver. The list of potential benefits can really bring an organization a lot of return on their initial investment, but that comes with a cost of deploying, maintaining, and developing the AIOps system over time. It also delivers ROI only when you have deployed it completely and correctly.

Developing Usable AIOps Metrics

With your deployments of AIOps from Chapter 4, you are running a base system, and it has been accumulating data from multiple sources. For example, if you use Splunk, you may have deployed it and been running it for perhaps three months gathering baseline data. If you are running ServiceNow with ITOM, you have collected data from all of your CIs. The point is, you are using a fully deployed system that is configured correctly, your data sources are trustworthy, and your AIOps system is ingesting them, making decisions and reporting on events accurately.

If you are using Splunk, you can use the built-in dashboards to generate the information you need. If you are using ServiceNow, you can build and use dashboards to provide the information you need. Exporting large amounts of data to use them in tools like Excel can be cumbersome, and many errors may result. Using tools like Crystal Reports and Yurbi (as examples) can help mine and provide visualization of data. When looking to develop state-of-the-art business intelligence (BI) data visualization, reporting, and metric development based on actionable data, these types of tools can provide many benefits beyond the standard dashboards in the AIOps tools. It should be said, however, that the AIOps tools I am reviewing in this book have large-scale enterprise-level BI function- ality within them and the power to conduct workflow automation and extensive metric development through the tools themselves. Although these other tools go way beyond the scope of this book and only aim to provide you with basic information for you to conduct more research on your own, it should be noted that these tools can provide benefits if you know them already, and if not, it's recommended that you research them.

Helpful Tools You Can Use

As noted, there may be times you need to take the data you have collected from your sources, or data sources themselves, and pipe it to a tool that can help you create a data visualization. While I will show you specific ways in the AIOps platforms to do this, there are some industry-leading tools you may need to use, or be confronted to use based on your organization. For example, many organizations today use a tool called Tableau to create data visualizations, but also actionable dashboards that help you work with that data.

First up is an older tool created by SAP called Crystal Reports (`crystalreports.com`). Although an old-timer in the world of BI, Crystal Reports is powerful and diverse and can handle just about anything you throw at it. Need customized data visualization, dashboards, and reports? This is your tool. Again, the tools you work with in the AIOps platforms (especially ServiceNow) are equally powerful, but for those who may choose a different AIOps tool or need more advanced output, have other reporting needs, or have the tools listed here and want to learn cross-functionality, you definitely have options. Crystal Reports is a BI tool developed by SAP that can be leveraged to provide deep insights into your data, deliver amazing-looking reports, and allow for customization through a myriad of available templates or building your own solutions. It is used to create custom reports based on a myriad of data sources that you can access with it. For example, it can provide help-desk statistics, KPI and CSF reporting data, and much more.

Another amazing tool that has been dethroning Crystal Reports for some time now is Tableau. Tableau (`www.tableau.com`) is a powerful and fast-growing data visualization tool used in the business intelligence industry. It is a desktop/server-based platform you can run in-house, or it can be a SaaS solution providing a web-based report visualization solution that provides much of the same analytics, data mining, BI, and customization as other tools. It is clearly a standout based on its ease of use compared to other platforms. Its format is simplified, and it can be programmed by those who spend some time learning the interface and available templates. Once you get the hang of it, you can be up and running quickly creating dashboards much like the one shown in Figure 5.4. Here you can see an executive dashboard highlighting much of what any operations platform tool will want to show you such as outages, incidents, time involved, problems, changes, requests, and so on.

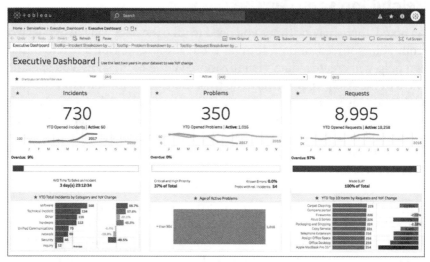

Figure 5.4: Using Tableau

Another valuable tool to consider for BI, ML, and AI is RapidMiner (rapidminer.com). The full package of RapidMiner Studio allows you to do BI, data visualization, and reporting, and it can help you build data models to test with. If you want to develop analytic processes, the templates and use cases available in the tool are top-notch. You can see an example of the tool and its available templates and use cases in Figure 5.5.

Lastly, you can use a tool similar to RapidMiner called Orange. Orange (orange.biolab.si) is an open-source data visualization, machine learning, and data mining toolkit. It features a visual programming frontend for explorative data analysis and interactive data visualization. Visual programming, development, and logic construction are strong points of Orange. Much like RapidMiner, you can use Orange for modeling. This is helpful when you want to understand what your data is telling you and how you can build better workflows around it. For example, if you have an influx of outages and want to try to develop an idea on how an AI engine may solve the problem, you can model it in Orange. You can also use the tool to help BI, reporting, and metric needs outside your AIOps toolset.

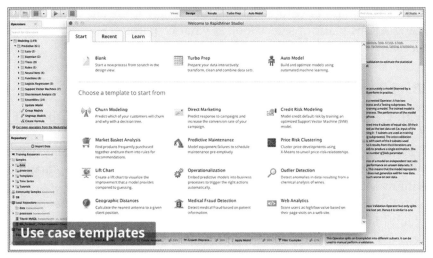

Figure 5.5: Using RapidMiner

TIP Don't stop there! There are hundreds of tools you can use. For example, there is another helpful tool called Domo (domo.com). This tool allows you to connect to data with more than 1,000 prebuilt APIs for data sources such as Salesforce, Google Big Query, and AWS, and do predictions, data visualization, reporting, and more using the built-in AI/ML tools. It even automatically normalizes data!

Gathering Usable Metrics

Gathering and developing usable output (metrics) for the enterprise can be a challenge in instances where you have an incomplete AIOps deployment, but if you have all of your data collected, systems deployed, and functionality in place, then you simply need to pull dashboards and reports (from templates) or build your own using the myriad of tools discussed in the previous section. That said, let's talk about why this is critical not only in healthcare but in any environment like sales forecasting, financials, or even trending a pandemic. Data is the source of all decision making, and if your data is bad, your decisions may not be accurate. The need for timely and complete data is paramount to developing what is needed for accurate decision making. Additionally, knowing how and when to pull data for metrics and reporting can save lives, keep systems running and operational, or simply save money.

To understand how to gather usable metrics for healthcare systems using AIOps platforms, let's look at what Dynatrace, Splunk, and ServiceNow with ITOM can provide out of the box.

Using Dynatrace

With Dynatrace, which we learned about in Chapter 3, the ability to develop and gather usable metrics is based on what you would like to report on. For example, you may need to report on the functionality of the system itself. You may need to report on the systems you are managing with the AIOps platform.

In this example, you experience impacts in your environment daily around the same time, and it causes clinical impact in your hospitals. Your assessment of the situation provides baseline data back from the operations center that you're getting some form of performance impact causing delays on key systems. These delays cause the clinician's impact that delays the providing of care.

Because of this, you want to review your AIOps system, pull the relevant information into a report looking at specific events, and trigger output, data points, and other metrical data to submit to the teams needed to fix the problem, or the leader who is requesting it. In Figure 5.6, you can pull within Dynatrace the processes that are reporting problems based on the output of a spiking or high-level CPU trigger.

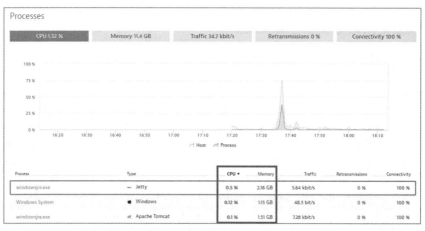

Figure 5.6: Dynatrace performance metrics

When you pull the relevant information, you can pivot it in a chart or print for review. Here you can report on the possible service performance metrics that are impacting your systems at that time and causing the degradation of service. As you can see from the performance metrics listed, many times CPU is the number-one impacted item in a system based on usage. For example, if the CPU is not able to handle what is asked of it, you will see it spike and even remain at a high level of usage, which can degrade the entire system and everything running on it. Another commonly used metric for performance is memory usage. Memory is consistently used by the system just like the CPU is and has a finite amount of available resources that, if maxed out to capacity, will also degrade the system's performance. Traffic is another one that can cause bottlenecks of data being requested where it cannot be provided fast enough, causing latency. Traffic or network traffic can be seen as a bottleneck as well, meaning that if the network card (NIC) or the port connection is overloaded and cannot handle the requests and what is asked of it, this can also cause a performance hit on the system. As you see, many of the metrics can show you where you need to add resources, power, or needed upgrades to the system to create an environment that can sustain what is asked of it.

Another valuable tool is to generate a custom chart. Aside from the amazing dashboards you saw in Chapter 3, you can pull and create custom charts based on usable data/metrics, as shown in Figure 5.7.

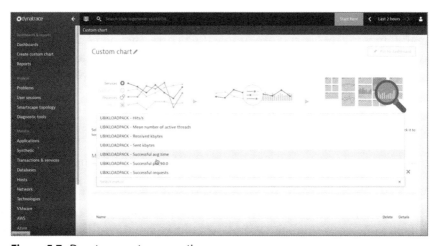

Figure 5.7: Dynatrace custom reporting

Most tools maintain canned reports and charts, and Dynatrace is no different. Here you can generate many common output requests. As noted, you can use Dynatrace to generate usable metrics, publish reports, create charts, or use the data to generate a report outside the tool.

Remember that this is just an example of what Dynatrace can do. This is by far nothing short of its massive power as an AIOps platform. The goal of this chapter is to prepare you for using your AIOps platforms in a way where they are using artificial intelligence (AI) and machine learning (ML) functions. To do so, the stepping-stone approach to get you to automation processes and workflows requires you to understand the basics of events, how those events are collected and reported in the AIOps platforms, and what you can do to retrieve them so you can validate whether automation is working.

To learn more, visit the website provided with each vendor to deep dive into the available (and sometimes infinite) functionality revolving around reporting, dashboard creation, metrics, data visualization, BI, and data analytics.

Using Splunk

Generating usable data metrics from Splunk can be done quite easily. Having usable metrics can help to determine issues, ongoing problems, and other events taking place in your environment. We also want our AIOps platform to be able to review what these problems are and report on them. Chapter 3 discussed Splunk as a platform to manage and maintain your infrastructure. If installed correctly and completely, the AIOps engine can be configured to automate responses (as discussed in Chapter 6) based on triggered events. In this chapter, we look at the reporting of those events.

Metrics can help any system administrator, systems engineer, network operator, help desk agent, manager, or other IT professional make good decisions on what is taking place in the environment. When using Splunk, you can review the events, faults, incidents, or other triggered events to gather metrics and pull reports. The data indexes are used to store metric data. You can access and show specific data by accessing them from the data indexes. As is discussed further in the next chapter, AIOps tools use automated workflows to harness the full power of AI; for now we will look at how to review what the systems are doing so we can either program the machine learning process into the tool or be able to see whether the AIOps platform is getting it right or wrong. Is the platform missing things? Are you experiencing outages and not seeing the tool respond correctly to it?

NOTE   You can configure an entire enterprise platform to manage your operations, but to ensure that you are getting the most bang for your buck, you need to do work such as analysis, review, metrics, and reporting to ensure that you are in fact getting the correct response from your systems.

Let's look at how Splunk can provide usable metric data when needed. To gather the information you need quickly, you can use metric storage retrieval commands such as mstats, mcatalog, and msearch on the metric data points in your data indexes. In the first example, I will use the mstats command to simply aggregate specific functions and data points like sum, average, and count to help identify (and isolate) issues from the aggregated data. Being able to correlate problems using these tools allows you to create the logic required to automatically resolve the issues based on what is found and identified as the root-cause problem. In Figure 5.8, mstats is used in a search function (of the data index) to create a visualization of processing power (CPU) and at what level it is functioning at.

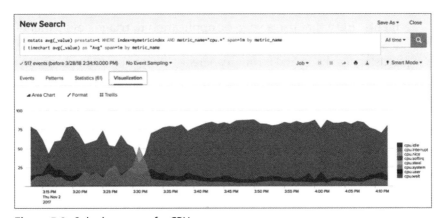

Figure 5.8: Splunk mstats for CPU

Figure 5.9 is another view of the same data index tool that shows on a timeline spikes rate hits with another way to see trends. Here, using the mstats query, you can investigate spikes of data that may go above the normal threshold or baseline and could cause (or are causing) an issue.

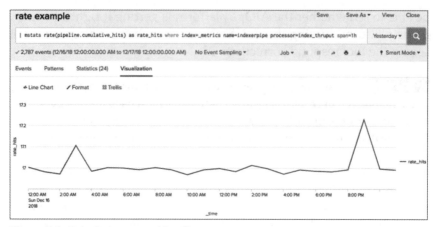

Figure 5.9: Splunk `mstats` with spikes

Here is a scenario where investigating how functionality that drops below an established baseline may be something you want to automate into an action, and knowing how to view this metric can help develop that action. In the following steps, I will lead you through a series of tasks that can be used to troubleshoot, analyze, and plan for handling performance issues.

1. You are experiencing an issue every day in your emergency departments (EDs) that use a specific application to triage new patients. It seems that at 8 p.m. there is a recurring slowdown of the tool causing it to hang and be nonresponsive. Follow-up attempts around 8:30 and 9 p.m. show better service.

2. The tool operates within normal parameters any other time of the day and has been found to be sensitive to latency.

3. You decide to investigate and find that there is a backup of the system that takes place at 8 p.m. and lasts for approximately 10 to 30 minutes every day. You have reviewed the application functionality, and there is no way to make adjustments to the application and no better time to do the backup. This investigation will include looking at the Splunk tools that were covered in the previous sections of this chapter to help look at statistical information on performance that can help you identify problems.

4. You find that adding a secondary node to the pool of servers hosting this application between 7 p.m. and 9 p.m. allows for more performance of the application to handle the backup window without issues occurring.

5. You create a workflow to automate this process, and it adds a server to the pool during this critical backup time.

Without investigating this problem, querying the data, reviewing the information, and understanding it, you will likely not be able to understand the logic behind AI and how it may handle this issue through a workflow. For example, the workflow states that a server will be added to the pool during this time to ease the service performance issue. What happens when the backup is light, is cancelled, or does not happen for some reason? It changes the logic. It also changes the workflow. If you have studied math, and specifically IT math, you can see that Boolean arguments will help to better understand how AI or ML may handle a workflow of this kind. IF the critical backup is running, THEN put an extra server in the pool to ease the pressure and provide better performance. IF the backup is not running, THEN do nothing. END. Simply put, without knowing how this works and instead letting the system just do it for you, you will not know how to handle false positives, incorrect processing of events, and many other factors that could cause difficulty in your ability to handle faults, problems, incidents and other issues that may arise.

Another tool you can use is `mcatalog`. In the New Search field you can query the index to report on events, patterns, and statistics (see Figure 5.10). The sampleEvent column will hold the information required such as a time-stamped event that may translate to a problem. For example, you may have a WAN link that is flapping or causing performance issues because it is disconnecting from the logical network.

NOTE   Splunk documentation indicates that `mcatalog` is an internal, unsupported, experimental command. Although that might call its reliability into question, many people use it without any noticeable, major problems.

Use the information in the catalog to review the events so that you can associate it with other events and attempt to correlate a problem. You can do this manually with the interface and log used in Figure 5.10.

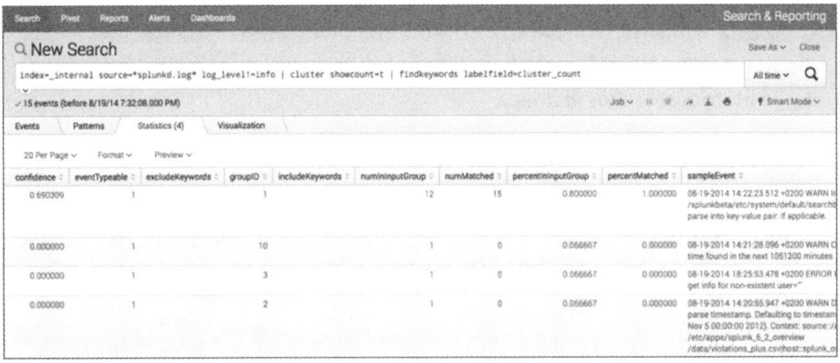

Figure 5.10: Splunk `mcatalog`

Part of understanding the data is being able to mine it, search for what you need, and then review your findings. If it isn't apparently clear, most of the large-scale systems host data in a database (or multiple databases or data warehouse structure) usually collected on enterprise storage platforms from companies such as Network Appliance or EMC. This data kept in large-scale enterprise-sized databases stored on these storage arrays and storage area networks (SANs) is quite large and, if set up to collect large amounts of data, can grow exponentially in size.

That said, part of your AIOps platform has to consider this as part of the needs of setting up a large system. Splunk stores much of its event data in a database, and you can use `msearch` to access and query it. Figure 5.11 shows the use of the ability to query, mine, search, and analyze needed data based on the saved history of the database.

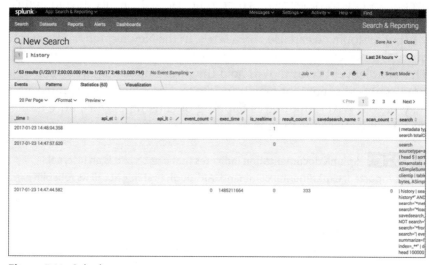

Figure 5.11: Splunk `msearch`

NOTE   For large-scale searches of metrics data, `msearch` can sometimes be slow to complete. Depending on your needs, `mstats` might be better for large metrics searches instead.

Now that we have looked at Splunk and how to manually use the system to probe for information and gather it for analysis, what about a dashboard where we can use most of this information or, better yet, see it in action when used with AI logic?

Since a metric is a single measurement at a specific point in time, what we would like to do in an enterprise platform like Splunk (or other platforms that use AI technology) is create the combined view of multiple data sources, events, and criteria to tell a story. Much like the storyboard concept discussed earlier in the "Information Technology Metrics" section, the use of a dashboard helps to create and visualize data in a way that tells the story of a problem, how it will be resolved, and if an issue occurring relating to an outage (as an example) was in fact restored to service. We would also like to generate reports based on that information and derive more metrics from historical views of this data to report on trends.

The Splunk Metrics Workspace is the interface that, when viewing Search and Reporting details, shows you metrics, datasets, alerts, and more. As you can see from Figure 5.12, you can pull reports, build dashboards, and do most if not all of the manual functions we just processed within the system. The tool is incredibly easy to use, is intuitive, and allows you a way to quickly aggregate data visually so you can act on real-time data as it is being processed.

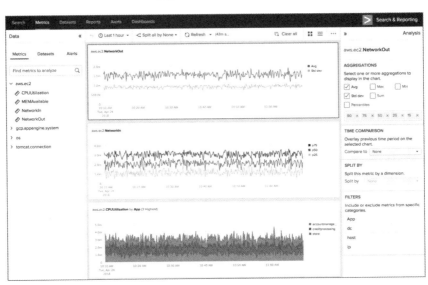

Figure 5.12: Splunk Metrics Workspace

The reason why you would want to use this toolset within the Splunk AIOps platform is for the ability to analyze the data you will automate actions on. Yes, metrics and understanding them are critically important to adding logic to actions that are going to create a successful outcome, and yes, it's important to be able to create reports for you and others to review, but first, a tool like this can provide you with insight. If your hospital staff is working on critical projects and cannot withstand an impact such as a down EMR tool, you can analyze the metrics to "predict" possible problems that may occur and be proactive with how they can be prevented.

This is one area where AI and ML start to get interesting: how you can predict an action based on what you believe may happen based on a trend. This is where I believe AIOps platforms must always be augmented with expert-level support staff that are analyzing the data, reviewing metrics and reports, and trying to be predictive with support. Most AIOps companies will say that AIOps augments humans, but this is a matter of perception. With ITIL and service operations, specifically problem management functions, the highest level of maturity you can gain in this area is with proactive problem management. Similarly to AI, proactive problem management is when a problem manager sees an active incident taking place (for example, a server performing badly), has seen in the RCA register that this problem has in fact happened before, and can act on what the corrective or preventative actions were in the past and restore service to the system (or proactively stop an impairment of service in the first place). This is where we see human intelligence rival AI in every way. So, how can we as AI programmers building an AIOps platform successfully build this logic into the platform? We will see as we work through the next two chapters that tools such as Splunk, ServiceNow, and others help create workflows that make sense.

The last part of understanding Splunk Metrics Workspace and how it can benefit you for AI, reporting, performance, and metrics is to know that it can help with real-time as well as older metric (stale) data for more current reportable information or for longer trend data. The way you may want to approach a data gathering effort like collecting server CPU performance would be to select a time range that specifically mapped to a problem area in the enterprise where you had a performance degradation. You can then apply filters that allow you to generate a report from related events within the captured log data so you can generate a shared view. The shared view can look at log data, events, and other captured metrical information and provide all data in one view for review. By doing so, you can combine data to get a more holistic view of an event or problem and what may be causing it. This is helpful when determining AI logic that can be used to help program solutions, automate workflow, and create actions that will be used to solve the issues that occur. To get this workspace, you can download it from Splunkbase, or, once you install an instance of Splunk (either Enterprise or Cloud), you will see it in the install set.

> **TIP**   Regardless of which product or tool you are using, make sure you get the concepts behind metrics, reporting, and understanding service performance. As a reminder, without a good background in what your systems are doing and how to review them, you may be in a situation where you need to provide automation help to your AIOps platform, and you cannot do that without knowing what is going on under the hood. Make sure you get this concept because you can apply it to every platform.

Using ServiceNow

With ServiceNow, you work on building AI reporting, metrics, service performance, and other relevant pieces of information from data sources and creating visualizations, reports, and dashboards on demand. ServiceNow is a large-scale IT service management (ITSM) tool that when loaded and used with all of its modules can help to provide a full-service management solution to include service desk, service performance, service operations, and many other service-related functions. With the IT operations module (ITOM), you can turn IT operations data into actionable results.

As your enterprise deployment of AIOps continues down the path to maturity, the use of a platform such as this can help to reduce the overhead of siloed data streams. It can also reduce the IT footprint by removing redundant tools from your portfolio that may all do the same thing and report on the same issues being discovered. Especially with the use of ServiceNow and ITOM, AIOps can use AI to help reduce that overhead. An example of how this can be accomplished would be to review your tool portfolio and find out what is duplication or what can be used to bolster another tool you may be using such as Splunk. ServiceNow works as an enterprise service management tool that can handle fault management and ticket generation for the help desk, but it may get its fault management information from Splunk as a trusted resource. You may have duplication with the ITOM module, but you may find enough value with Splunk through the use of their detailed tools and performance stats to use both simultaneously.

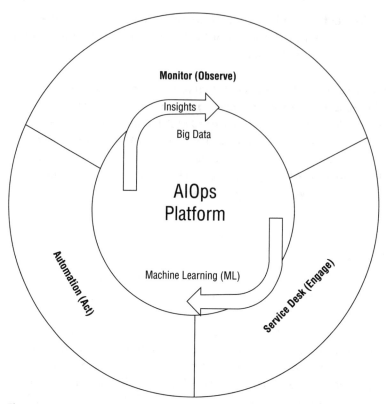

Figure 5.13: AI for ServiceNow ITOM

First, you should know how ServiceNow works with all of the components in your enterprise to create a useful system that can help bring together all of the components you will want to report on. Figure 5.13 shows the cycle where AIOps is at the center of all your other systems. This is the story we want to build as we deploy ITOM AIOps so that you can in fact develop usable KPIs, metrics, reports, and other visualizations from actionable data. You can also see that in the center of the AIOps engine is big data, which is the culmination of all the data in your enterprise. It should be part of a master data management (MDM) program to ensure that all data is clean, compliant, and manageable. It is also extremely large and normally associated with many large data sets that can be used as a whole to produce patterns, trends, and associations once analyzed.

Other components that make up the engine are the revolving and cyclical functions of continuous insights that help build the three pillars of engagement, observation, and action. In the next chapter, we will cover action with automation. All of this brings business value to the table, which is what you are looking to gain with your AIOps deployment.

You provide the business value through continuous insights of big data through your AIOps platform. This comes from commonly used metrics that are derived from the system, the use of this data to storyboard, and then the deployment of automation to help build on what you want the system to do. Figure 5.14 highlights many of the functions that allow ITOM to bring that functionality to life.

Figure 5.14 shows the storyboard concept as well; however, this is more of a flowchart schematic that shows how the functionality works to provide the data required for action. Here you can see alerts that are collected and filtered, marked, and used within the machine learning components of the system to allow for anomaly detection, alert correlation, and discovery and root-cause analysis. Through all of this, automation can be used to allow for actions.

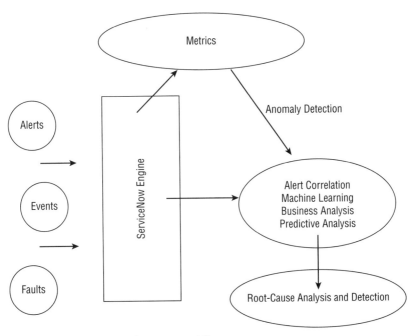

Figure 5.14: ServiceNow business workflow

In Figure 5.15, the data becomes more actionable based on the use of the data. For example, now that you have actionable data that has been refined by the AIOps platform, workflows can be created to provide for business processing, usage by business services, and much more. For the sake of driving the need and use of reporting, all of this data can be reported on and better understood to provide for the automation workflows on actionable data. Here you can see that customers, employees, partners, clinicians, vendors, and internal IT staff can work with advanced machine learning functions to include self-service functions all the way to predictive incident management. When we look at ServiceNow and ITOM, the use of the collaboration of processes through a modular approach allows for a building block deployment of full functionality to include ML at all levels of the workflow.

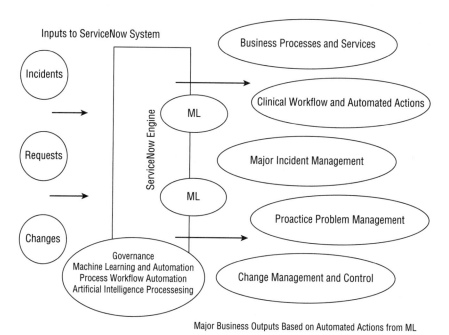

Figure 5.15: Business services and ML

Lastly, through the use of the AIOps platform, its collection of services, and how it builds on the collected data, there is a myriad of other platforms that can in fact work with ServiceNow as a whole to provide a large-scale deployment of AI solutions on- and off-premise, with the use of a full cloud or hybrid cloud solution or with the use of other operations platforms to help provide that service. You can see this in Figure 5.16 where the connection of all systems provides one large-scale AIOps platform that can be leveraged together.

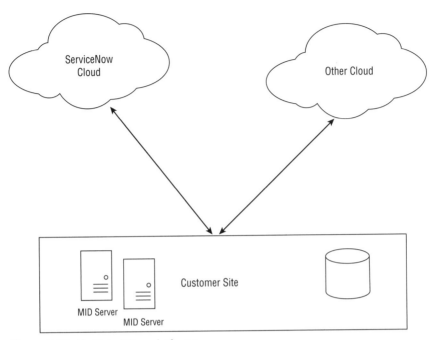

Figure 5.16: Multiple AIOps platforms

Once you know how you will lay out your platform, what story you want to tell, what functions you need to deploy, and how that will relate to actions and workflows, you can move to pull key metrics and reports and view service performance for next steps on how you want to deploy ServiceNow to call on that data and use it through automation.

The next step is in Figure 5.17 and what will start to bridge the gap between understanding the storyboard, the layout of the system, what it is collected, what it's connected to, and what it is reporting. Once you measure the performance, you can start to derive what actions the system will take. Although I will focus on this in the next chapter, as I mentioned with Splunk and the other tools I have covered in this chapter, if you do not know how to lay out the system and what it is telling you without automation, you will be hard-pressed to deploy automation or, in the best case, let the platform automate it for you.

In Figure 5.17, you can see how ServiceNow dashboards can be used to create automation. The key to success here is to have an ITSM system like ServiceNow with clean data through the use of CIs, a CMDB, and other trusted sources of data you can rely on. Here in this example, a workflow is developed based on understanding data variables that, once connected via the storyboard, will allow for actions to be taken.

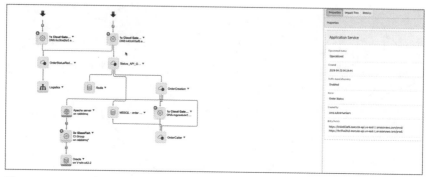

Figure 5.17: Translating to workflow

For example, in this example cloud sources of Oracle are used and can be seen with the visualizer down to the service view level. This will highlight all CIs that are associated with this service and how it may or may not be impacted. For example, if one part of the service is impaired like the database, it will report on that and likely send out an alert. This may or may not impair the entire service. ServiceNow will report on this by cutting a ticket and engaging a resource like the help desk. Although this is what commonly may be done, there are a lot of factors that must be considered. For example, the database may have a secondary node that, once it identifies that it has been compromised, may enact the secondary node to take over the service. This may only cause a disruption in service momentarily and, through the use of automated functions like a failover to a new node, may immediately restore service and lower the ticket status from a priority one incident (very high) to a priority three, which means that a repair is still required. The service is up and running, but the service as a whole (as shown in the visualizer) is impacted. AI not only brings actionable insight to network operators in problem resolution but also provides predictive problem analysis, essentially solving problems before they become problems.

Regardless of whether you are using ServiceNow or another platform, there are several factors and concerns you should keep in mind:

- Great care goes into the design and strategy of a good AIOps platform.
- You need to understand how your business works at every level that your AIOps platform may integrate.
- A high level of understanding of current IT systems is a requirement.

- When selecting the AIOps platform, you should have a scope created to understand what you want to accomplish based on the previous three bullets.

- Once you have an understanding of what you want to deploy and how, you need to understand the why, as has been discussed throughout this chapter.

- You should storyboard what story you want to tell with the data you are collecting to help develop the workflows needed for automation. This is the foundation of successful AI and ML operations.

- By knowing how to report on data, understand metrics, create KPIs and CSFs, and plan on your ingested data, you can create actions that make sense.

- Knowing that the systems are doing what they are intended for allows you to know whether AI is working and whether AI is working correctly for you (solving problems, not creating them and/or not missing things).

- No system is installed without a support system to manage, monitor, tune, and analyze it.

Lastly, no system of this size is plug and play. You simply do not run setup.exe and have an AIOps system that is fully automated and reduces IT costs. I will address this further when I discuss common KPIs, metrics, and clinical concerns that drive the need for healthcare IT, AIOps, and a good understanding of how that translates to clinical operations.

Clinical and IT Metrics and Collective Actions

In this section, I want to give you the knowledge to tie everything together so that you can build on your "why." The goals of AIOps are to reduce problems, make life easier, and create a way for actions to be learned and automated by the system. It's simplistic sounding, but not always easy to create, particularly when trying to successfully deploy AIOps in a critical environment such as healthcare.

With the backdrop of a health system deploying AIOps into their environment, it helps to make sense of how clinician needs, metrics, KPIs, and other dependencies play into the needs and wants of clinicians who are stakeholders in the AIOps plan. Figure 5.18 shows the gamut of clinical operations that all require support from IT operations.

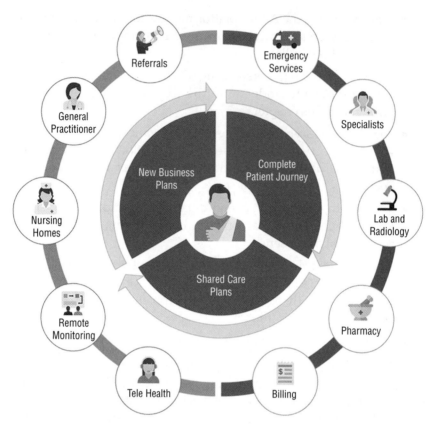

Figure 5.18: Clinical use of IT

The clinical functions as outlined in Figure 5.18 show how the patient is impacted by clinical services that surround them. All these services (to include any and all data about the patient) are contained within IT systems. Therefore, it would be safe to conclude that any aspect of the clinical plan, treatment, or any part of the patient experience is in fact covered by technology at some point. Whether it is the care provider using systems to access records, input patient information, send labs, request medications, send prescriptions, access other parts of the patient medical record, connect with a specialist, consult another doctor via telemedicine, connect any part of this to patient billing, or send out a referral, every single aspect is covered with healthcare IT. The reason this becomes important is that all of this maps to systems that are being maintained by operations groups that need to keep each and every aspect of the infrastructure and the systems that reside on it healthy and available. All these aspects can be covered by both clinical and IT metrics. They become a collective action, and although they are separate metric and reporting functions, they do in fact line up when showing the bigger picture of an enterprise and how well it is functioning.

Developing metrics should be done separately; however, they should be considered together at some point. When you look at sample healthcare metrics, reports, KPIs, CSFs, and performance data, you can see the results of how well your business is running. If your IT systems are not able to maintain a stable environment, this will immediately impact every single metric in the clinical workflow. For example, if you consider available beds in a hospital, if rooms have systems that are down in them, this may impact the available room. If an operating room is unable to perform because of failed IT system, this may impact doctor block time. There are so many ways that these metrics intersect and impact each other, and as a leader in the organization, you need to consider them. When it comes to AIOps platforms and the ability to sell the ROI of high availability due to the use of correct workflows to keep systems up and running, if you're unable to show that in both IT and clinical metrics, you may have to uncover why. The answer may be that you are not aligning them and they are not in sync to show similar aspects of up or down time, or it is possible that you are seeing these issues but cannot map them to a failed system because the metrics and reporting are not aligned. Either way, having an AIOps platform and showing ROI for it should require you to marry up the two sets of metrics or show a clear impact of ROI across both sets of reports when you are running a fully functional system that you know is making an impact in your environment.

The next step would be to develop new KPIs that show the benefits of AIOps and the platform you are using. MTTR should not be the only KPI that you find valuable. You can also take this moment to develop your own. Yes, KPIs are in fact something you can develop that help to show specifically what your organization finds valuable and what it can and cannot live without. For example, whatever results (both positive and negative) that can be derived from data to show an organization how it can evaluate its activities could prove useful.

To develop a new KPI, you can map an objective (clinical bed availability) that your stakeholders agree is important and include data that can be used to prove that the results of the objective are positive or negative. What is the threshold number (metric) that gives you a good outcome or a negative one? What makes it actionable? For one, if you find that key systems that may impact the available beds (for example, an RFID chip malfunction to track beds) seems to be a constant issue, then the review of those systems may be what needs to be evaluated and measured. To keep the KPI in a positive state, use your AIOps platform to pull metrics, reports, and dashboards on those key systems and build workflow to help keep them maintained. This may not always be the case. You may have a defect that an operations platform that tracks and handles events just cannot solve. This is where problem management comes in and creates a corrective action. Then, if you find that the system is still defunct because of an action that is in fact fixable or maintainable by AIOps, create automation to solve the problem. Once you have that in place, after a specific period of time (perhaps one month), review the metric and see where it is trending. If you find that the RFID technology is remaining stable and that bed availability remains high, you may have a positive outcome for your metrics, and you have met your KPI. As in Figure 5.19, you can see that all data will interconnect from the bedside so that clinicians can quickly use all relevant information as it is needed.

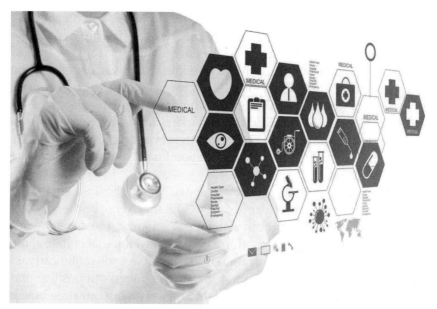

Figure 5.19: Readily accessing clinical data

There are many, many other KPIs; however, this should be enough to give you an idea of how all of it ties together nicely with showing ROI for your AIOps platform. You know if you are hitting goals and if you are meeting your KPIs; it's that simple. You know you are hitting those goals if your AIOps platform is the reason why you are able to maintain high availability of service performance. This is the ROI. As a reminder, the tie-in to healthcare is easy to remember: the ROI is met when your KPI (or metric) is met when hitting a clinical goal is accomplished. Another benefit is when you are able to tie it to patient satisfaction and positive outcomes on the clinical side. Building better outcomes through data analysis is but one major step why many healthcare systems are looking at AIOps among other analytics and intelligence solutions.

> **NOTE**   Healthcare has taken a giant leap into informatics. With the use of big data, the analysis of that data, and the ways to use the data to create positive outcomes, it's no wonder we are looking at total convergence. A word to the wise: remember that all of this convergence creates complexity. This is why understanding the story, what the data is telling you, and how to work with the data to better understand it is critical to AI, ML, and data visualization.

Usable Healthcare AIOps Dashboards

Service desk tie-ins, reporting examples, being able to quickly pull up and use data, reviewing patient information, and having real-time analysis of critical data are where we will be heading into the future of AI, ML, and specifically AIOps platforms. Increasing service delivery through performance is a goal of every leader in every health system. We are sitting on a large amount of data that can help to provide for better care. We just need to know how to leverage it. Although traditional AIOps systems are used to keep operations up running and IT systems available through automation and workflows, this does not mean it does not become part of the bigger picture in any industry it supports. As you can see in Figure 5.20, the key to high availability of clinical data comes from the ability to immediately use the technology by the clinicians as they are working in real time.

This means that if you wanted to provide care, and, for example, there is a problem sending a blood lab to the laboratory or a problem getting meds up from the pharmacy, you can quickly use a mobile tablet to open a service desk ticket to get a technician working on the problem immediately. A better solution is a proactive one. What if you can have AIOps identify that the system is not working before the clinician can report it? This is where we want to go with the future of AIOps platforms especially within healthcare. If the patient is never impacted by a system that is down or unavailable, patient care via technology would be seamless, and the clinical staff can worry about clinical matters and not why the computer doesn't work.

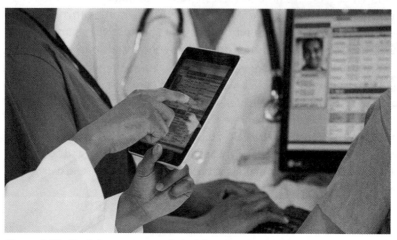

Figure 5.20: Real-time access to clinical data is supported by AIOps.

AI functionality with machine learning components could see that the lab system is down, cut a ticket to get a tech working on it, call out to an on-call engineer for immediate priority one support, failover to a working node that may be performance degraded due to an oversaturated switch port, and report to the clinician's handheld that the system is running at 100%.

CAUTION   Because of the complications of security, PHI/PII, HIPAA compliance, PCI, and many other restrictions, it is important that you review all of your company's security policies, HR and business policies, and any other policies that state what you can or can't do with data prior to moving forward into configuring advanced automation or workflows.

Summary

So, as we started this chapter with a quote by Aristotle stating that excellence is never an accident and happens to be the result of high intention, sincere effort, and intelligent execution, such are the efforts of deploying an intelligent AI solution for your healthcare operation. It represents wise choices such as what tools to use, what story you want to tell with your data, how you want that data to represent action, and finally, as the next chapter will explore, how that data can be used to create actions that present good return on investment and reduction of incidents, outages, and issues. The process of service reporting is a choice but a wise choice nonetheless, especially if your chosen destiny is to have a highly functioning AIOps platform making good decisions based on clean data that it has ingested. In the next chapter, you will learn about workflows, automation, how to act on data, and what that translates to in an IT healthcare environment.

AIOps and Automation in Healthcare Operations

"Number 5 is alive."

—Short Circuit

Once AIOps has been deployed and you are working with a fully operational tool, what more can it do for you? How do you really reap the return on investment (ROI) of a system that takes advantage of artificial intelligence (AI)? By setting up workflows, processes, and automation functionality within the toolset, you can begin to see how the AIOps system can really make an impact. Automation is the intelligence that a system will use to create actions based on the workflow set up and designed by process engineers. Once the system can "learn," it can be used to create a workflow based on use case, scenarios, common outcomes, and more. To get the most benefit, you need to have a fully configured system (covered in Chapters 1–5) and other components such as a CMDB and trusted sources of data providing you with usable actions. In this chapter, we will look at all of the variables associated with automation, workflow engineering, process engineering, and getting AI and ML to work for you.

This chapter discusses how healthcare systems can utilize their AIOps platform in a way that reduces outages, increases service performance and availability, and improves overall system usage for clinical functions.

Automation, Workflow, Process, and Intelligence Design

When it comes to intelligent system design, there are many concepts that need to be considered prior to deployment. In this chapter, one of the main concepts to deploying AIOps platforms is to understand the goals of automation, workflows, process handling, machine learning, and how artificial intelligence concepts all tie together. When you first deploy your AIOps platform, it is basically an event management (fault management) platform that after you handle population (perhaps through discovery), you get alerted to conditions and thresholds that are exceeded or tripped via settings you configure. From there, what does the platform do? Cut a ticket? Send an alert? Contact on-call teams to handle the alert? Try to self-heal? All of these concepts need to be understood but also strategized as part of your AIOps platform deployment.

Once you have these concepts worked out and they are understood, you can begin the project of configuring the actions that the platform will take when these conditions are met and what the platform will do when they are needed. For example, if a threshold is exceeded like a disk quota and we are going to run out of disk space on a system, there are multiple things that can happen, and you may want to design the system to do them in a specific order. You may want to first have a ticket cut and or an alarm sent in tandem to alert the on-call person that the threshold has been breached. From there, you can take and call out other actions, or the system itself can start to automate actions. When AI has become part of the process after a considerable amount of time learning about the system, it too can take actions based on the disk quota being exceeded. Although this is but one simple example, there are literally thousands of examples that can be derived from this one example, and those are the concepts we will cover in this chapter from the basics of automation strategy to complete process and workflow design as well as how AI will function in a completely self-healing system.

Designing the Framework for Automation

In this chapter, we will look at the importance of AI and ML and at how automation and workflow process engineering play a large role in your strategy, deployment, and system performance outcomes. By understanding automation, you will be better positioned to make decisions on how it will be used within your system to complete the goals you set out to achieve. A wide range of goals is possible, including improving users' experience, establishing self-healing solutions, using self-reporting, providing alerting solutions to improve resolution time, and more. Design workflow and process engineering can be examined to ensure that all the automation, rules, event responses, and programming put in place work properly and reduce the chance of error. Deploying the foundation and all that comes with it like CMDB, configuration items, trusted sources, and other key infrastructure can help in making sure that your AIOps platform has all of the foundational items needed to ensure that automation can not only take place, but take place correctly.

Service mapping is another important function that allows for you to use automation to address issues such as outage scenarios that affect a service. An example would be to service-map an EMR platform. If the EMR has an outage, the backend infrastructure is mapped out in a way so that the service mappings know that, for example, a database may be impacted, which could disrupt the use of the EMR. One way of handling this would be for an automated function to fail over to a secondary node. Once your services are designed and mapped and your AIOps platform is configured with automation and rules, you can test the system for accuracy. Lastly, it is important to monitor and troubleshoot issues that occur with automation to ensure the best outcomes. First, let's look at what automation is and why it's imperative to the AIOps platform working properly.

Understanding Automation

Artificial intelligence, machine learning, and automation all work together. There is a growing need to remove the repetitive steps from managing an operations platform and systems for information technology. Automation is one of the ways in which repetitive tasks can be streamlined and made easier by technology. Today, automation works with AI and ML and even more so with new platform-based enterprise systems like AIOps platforms. Tools like Splunk, ServiceNow, and others have the ability to take the information they are collecting in their large databases, combine that with what has been learned, and automate a response based on either what they are told to do or what they have learned to do.

Automation in its most basic form is nothing more than taking a workflow and finding a way to streamline it with processes that remove manual effort from the equation. For example, if I had a software update I needed to run for 100 machines across my enterprise, either I could have technicians install all of these instances separately or I could use a tool like Microsoft's Group Policy to push the update out to the machines, thereby automating it and saving time, effort, and manpower. This is a simplistic view of automation but probably one of the most common forms of it in IT today. Software distribution has almost become entirely automated, making the care and feeding of desktop systems much easier to maintain and keep updated.

In AIOps platforms, creating automated workflows can be done very easily when you have all of the requirements satisfied, the system deployed and designed correctly, and the correct monitoring of the outcome of the automated efforts. In the previous chapters, I discussed the need and importance of deploying a complete system. In this chapter, I explore the importance of the rest of the foundational items that have been discussed but are not crucial for automated efforts to take place, such as a configuration management database (CMDB). In the next sections of this chapter, I will outline what CMDB is and why it is important for automation to be successful.

Improved User Experience

When it comes to AIOps platforms, healthcare clinical outcomes being made better by AIOps, and improving efficiency, quality control, and better uptime for critical systems, automation can bring your AIOps system to life. Improving the clinical user experience can be made better simply by ensuring that key systems like the EMR are up and running and stay that way. For example, if you have an AIOps platform like Splunk running and managing your network infrastructure, it is possible to set up automation so that when the tool is doing standard event management functions like responding to a triggered event, it can be set up to handle a response to that event. For example, a network port has been opened and it's causing a Spanning Tree loop. It may be possible to have the system configured to automate the use of a different port when that condition arises. The AI functionality would be useful because, if that condition arises, the most common scenario identified from the learned data that has been collected thus far would be to move to a different port based on ML's ability to evaluate previous situations that have taken place and those that resulted in a positive solution. The concept that needs to be understood is that AI would either recommend to the Networks Operations team that a loop was occurring and make the recommendation that a new port be used or trigger an automated process that switches the port without human intervention. Here is where we see the benefits of both automation and AI being part of solving the problem within the system. All of this intelligence on the backend is used to make sure that the technology remains up and functional so that the EMR system stays up and responsive. This ensures the clinical staff have continued access to the EMR and allows them to be clinicians and not spend time on making calls to the help desk to fix these issues or on downtime procedures documenting their work on paper.

How AIOps can be automated to improve experience is just a bigger picture of the clinical example I just used. For example, the need to keep the network stable, the EMR up and running, and/or desktop systems patched and updated contributes to an improved end-user experience. It also reduces the need for an IT footprint to handle redundant and/ or repetitive tasks. Defining repeatable tasks can be done by simply looking at the processes you currently have in your organization and doing a process improvement, analysis, and review session. By looking at how your current processes are managed, you can learn a lot about what is wasteful about them. Further, by setting up governance around it, reviews, and data metric reports (discussed in Chapter 5), you can really put a good project plan together to help remove waste, build automated workflows, design them, test them, and deploy them with your AIOps solution.

> **TIP**   As will become apparent in the "Designing Workflow and Process Engineering" section, you will need to put work into understanding what you have before you go and fix it. AIOps and other large-scale enterprise applications are normally not plug and play (meaning that you plug it in and you get what you want out of it immediately). Many times, the best deployments come from a dedicated team working through all of the items we discuss in this book to make sure that your deployment of your AIOps platform not only delivers what is expected but also overdelivers. The next section on designing workflow will be important to understand as we move into designing processes that can be automated and intelligently handled by AI.

Designing Workflow and Process Engineering

Designing a workflow is as simple as understanding what is being done already and then mapping it. Figure 6.1 can be used as an example of how you can put together a process workflow chart and decision tree using swim lanes to help break down what a process looks like and how it operates.

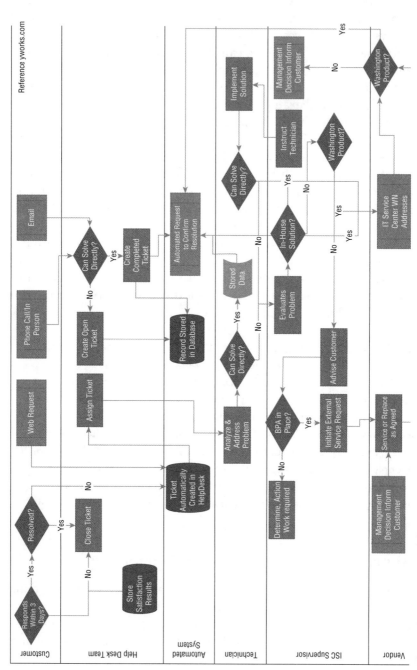

Figure 6.1: Process workflow map

Note that Figure 6.1 is a simple example of a help-desk workflow. It helps to paint the picture of understanding that any other process is going to look similar. Here are the key takeaways of viewing a process of this type:

- The process map is usually outlined with swim lanes where each "lane" represents a group or person that handles the task, process block, or decision that takes place.

- The groups are all the stakeholders of the process. For example, the process may be "how to handle a help desk ticket" as an example, but you may have more groups involved other than the help desk. You have the customer or client that calls in a ticket. You may have different levels of escalation inside and outside your main group, such as higher support tiers of engineers who handle issues, or different groups that handle technology services altogether. Either way, each lane must include all groups involved in the process.

- The process itself follows a mathematical function such as Boolean math. For example, IF someone does a specific thing, THEN this will be what happens or what needs to happen, ELSE there is some other alternate thing that will happen.

- The process needs to have a clear start and end point to it so that there is no confusion when adjustments to the process need to be made. There can be subprocesses that align and some that cross-connect to your process. However, it is important to divide up and compartmentalize process functions as much as possible for the sake of maintenance and handling.

- You can make a process for just about anything. Understanding how to lay out a process is what will get you up to speed on how to get better at doing them.

At this point, we have discussed process engineering functions; how to lay out, design, and map these functions in a tool; and how to document them. We can now move into finishing the foundational design for creating an automation function for your AIOps platform. We can also discuss snapping in these processes so that they will provide you with the automation needed to streamline your efforts, make your response quicker, improve your uptime, and capitalize on the other benefits to AI, ML, and using automation.

A WORD ABOUT SIX SIGMA

There are many process engineering systems available and overall programs to help find inefficiencies in your processes. You can use a system like Six Sigma to remove waste, defects, and other unwanted or ineffective tasks from your process. Although there is no "one-size-fits-all" approach to what system works best for reviewing and fixing processes, Six Sigma and Six Sigma Lean (a consolidated version) allow you to take a problem with a process and put it through a Define, Measure, Analyze, Improve, and Control (DMAIC) process to mathematically identify through statistical analysis what could be creating waste. However, way beyond the scope of this book, it should be noted that the best process automation comes from the best functioning processes without automation.

DMAIC can be used to create a cycle that once completed will allow you to understand a process from start to finish and, like the swim lanes, understand all parties involved and how they relate to that process. For example, one of the tools is a SIPOC chart that looks at the supplier and customer and all the inputs and outputs to each part of a process.

TIP   A tool such as Microsoft Visio can be used to help create process workflows, swim lane charts, and other process engineering design charts that can help you lay out and better understand what your processes look like and all of their inputs and outputs.

Process engineering can sometimes be looked at as decision-making (auto-enabled) or decision trees much like when you call a company and are asked a long list of questions prior to speaking with an agent. Your process may also look like this and may not be beneficial to automation. For example, if you have too many decisions that need to be made, automation will become more complex, and if powered by ML and AI, it could be contaminated by bad data and wrong decisions made by the system.

Quality Control and Assurance

Quality control and assurance functions need to be in place so that processes and workflows that are automated can be validated that they are still functional, relevant, providing service, and not injecting errors. Quality can be assessed many ways. You can spot-check a process and test it for accuracy. One of the ways you can do this is by running the process in a test lab or in a controlled fashion. When you do this, you need to record the process and its results so that you can assess on a weighted scale if your process works well or not. Does it create the anticipated outcome?

For example, if your process was to deploy updates to software on machines that needed it, how would that look from a process inspection standpoint when providing quality assurance? It may look something like this:

1. If all desktops with a specific operating system are online and available, check the database and see whether they have the updates we are looking to deploy already installed.

2. If those desktops do have the updates installed, do not reinstall them. If the desktops don't have the updates installed, install them.

3. After the updates are successfully installed on all of the necessary desktops, make sure that there are no missed systems by scanning for the updates and reporting on any desktops that don't have them.

This is a simple view of this automated process, but there are many things that could go wrong. For example, what about systems that are not in the database? What about systems that were installed incorrectly and were not part of the deployment group? How about if you find out that there are systems with different versions of operating systems that do not allow for this patch to be installed? What if the patch got corrupted on 20% of the machines it was installed on? What if the patch caused other problems? I can really go on and on here, but the point is that you need to keep an eye on spot-check automation, perform some quality checks, and ensure that it's doing what it's intended to do. This is why it is generally good to use a CMDB, which will be discussed later in this chapter.

Foundational and Required Design Items

As we design the automation for our system, there are some important design items you need to consider. For example, as I have mentioned in earlier chapters, understanding the storyboard for your deployment goes a long way in deploying it correctly. If you know what you want your system to look like, how you want it to function, and what actions you want it to take, then designing the event management and handling and automating events will take place in a more simplistic fashion.

Similarly, when deploying systems such as Splunk, ServiceNow ITOM, or other platforms, you need to have trusted data sources for your inputs.

A fully deployed AIOps solution means that you have the system deployed and configured correctly and it's collecting data or reviewing trusted data sources such as a centralized database of information or other central repository of data. Most likely, this will be something your entire enterprise will leverage such as a configuration management database (CMDB). The CMDB is nothing more than a database that stores the information about your system assets and does so in a way that uses markings on those configuration items (CIs) to utilize a trusted data source of owned and used assets. This is also considered part of an IT asset management (ITAM) deployment. The reason why this is so important to have as part of an automation solution is that it's literally the backbone of all of the services that you will map and create actions for. Service mapping is how you use the CMDB data to create relationships between services, assets, data, and other owned information. Figure 6.2 shows an example of the CMDB in.

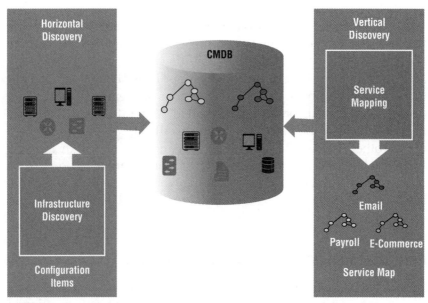

Figure 6.2: The CMDB, CIs, and service mapping

Now that you have a CMDB, the next step is to make sure that it is populated. You can do this by setting discovery or manually entering key data. Now, this may go beyond the scope of this book, which is to design and deploy an AIOps solution in a healthcare environment, but the use of the CMDB cannot be overstated. Remember what I said earlier in the book about ROI. If you sell your leadership on the ability to do some type of artificial intelligence with your operations service platform, you need the system to be complete, and it has to be able to make good decisions on the events that take place. The only way that this can happen is by making sure that you have a clean source of data to make decisions on and that the actions taken are reasonably based on that data. Similarly, your organization's goals and your service desk's top problems need to be addressed as well. An example would be to consider having an AIOps platform enabled to ensure that if an EMR is unavailable, the AIOps platform can do something about it using some form of AI. That translates to automation functions whether established by you as an architect or done by the system itself as part of ML. Either way, you need to make sure that your foundational items are designed correctly, and that comes down to service mapping.

Service mapping is another important function that allows for automation to take place correctly based on outage scenarios that affect a service so that if you have some type of problem, the automated features act accordingly and do what you want them to do.

There are many ways to service map. However, the two you will see utilized here are vertical and horizontal. In Figure 6.2 you can see that no matter what source of building relationships occurs, as long as they wind up in the CMDB as a trusted source and that source shows a complete picture of the service, all of its assets, and configuration items, you can move to the next step, which would be to configure automated functions. In Figure 6.3 you can see an example of horizontal discovery and how relationships are developed.

Horizontal Discovery Relationships

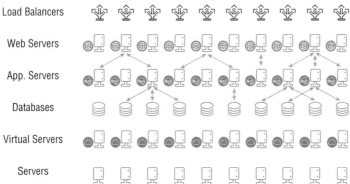

Figure 6.3: Horizontal discovery

Here we can see the components that may make up the underlying systems and infrastructure that may make up the EMR. An EMR can be a large deployment in a health system. An EMR can include and be supported by many components such as servers, routers, switches, VMs (virtual servers), load balancers, associate databases, frontend web servers . . . the list goes on and on. If you are running a large EMR platform, you may have thousands of subsystems that compose the EMR system. That said, you would look at the entire EMR as one collective service and consider all of its components and infrastructure to be part of it. Think of it like this: if we do a horizontal discovery, you can see that certain web servers communicate with specific application (app) servers. Those are configured or mapped to specific datasets housed in certain databases. They may be part of a specific data warehouse housed on a storage area network (SAN). Those DB systems may be physical servers or virtual machines. Although I simplified the horizontal discovery and only gave you a small glimpse of how deep it can go (it can go much deeper), you can start to see why this discovery is critical to automation and AI.

If you want the EMR to self-heal based on some type of outage (for example, a VM may become corrupted), your service is impacted, and you can see the event trigger for an impacted VM that can cause an outage to that service. You can create a rule (or a rule can be configured by the system in the form of an action based on learned data) to snapshot the VM or use a backup VM that may be online.

TIP   You should start to realize the importance of the CMDB and service mapping as critical to an event or fault management system in use today. You may have the EMR service mapped, but you may also have other service mappings, such as another critical system or application. For example, if your labs run on a different system or your billing on another, you can see what that would mean if they all used the same database that suddenly becomes unavailable. This means that three critical services could be impacted by one outage. Make sure that you understand your services and service mappings and have your enterprise understood, documented, and mapped as much as possible before deploying an AIOps platform because the data from these systems could really help create the automation functions needed to realize the true benefits of your AIOps investment.

Vertical service mapping is another approach. As we saw with horizontal service mapping, the CIs are used to create the discovery through the ServiceNow (SN) discovery module. Vertical service mapping can be seen as pure service mapping. As shown in Figure 6.4, you can map the specifics of the service such as telling the system that specific systems are part of a service, and it allows that information to help create the full map of the service. In this example, you know that the mappings are specifically depicted by the engineer to make the service map. Horizontal discovery can use the discovery module to run a scan and by giving it an IP range to work with. So, if your EMR runs on the 10.2.10.0 network, it will discover all of the connected items in that range. This can be thought of as the service discovery process, as shown in Figure 6.5.

Vertical Service Mapping Discovery

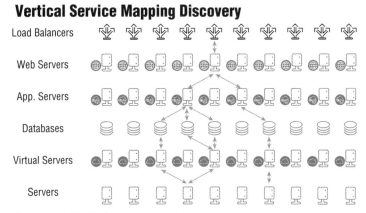

Figure 6.4: Vertical service mapping

Service Discovery Process

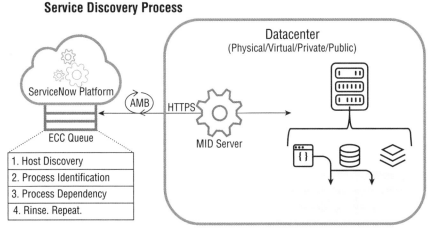

Figure 6.5: Service discovery process

Service discovery is critical to having a complete picture of a service that will be mapped. Again, do not lose sight of the goal. We want the

AIOps platform to be able to know what a service looks like so it can have a complete picture of all the dependencies. A database that has an indexing need or a corruption problem can cause disruption in your clinicians' work because they cannot run labs and perform their work. A bigger problem is the IT team not knowing why this happens, what to do, or where to start. This would especially be the case when having spent major capital on an AIOps platform that is nothing more than a glorified fault management system sending alerts and cutting tickets.

The answer is an intelligent system run by those who have correctly designed it to act by manual or dynamic intervention to respond to these faults or events with an action of restoring service. It does this by having a complete picture of what that service is and the underlying infrastructure that supports it. Once you have a complete mapping, you can see dependency views that allow you to visualize what is broken and what it will impact, but most importantly, the AIOps system can be used to take action against these dependencies and try to resolve the problem.

Figure 6.6 shows the service mapping process where information is passed from one point to the other and collected by the system in a way that allows the service to be built and saved by the platform. The process will start with an entry point that is some type of connection to the systems, services, and other assets on the network. For example, I mentioned earlier that an IP range can be specified. You can also put a service entrance point for discovery. For example, there may be a URL or web link used to gain access to a system or service.

The Service Mapping Process

- **Entry Point**
  - URL, connection parameters, etc.
- **Host detection**
  - Connection to target machine, discovery CI information
- **Process Identification**
  - Identify the application based on information from entry point
- **Connection Discovery**
  - Discover configured connection to other applications

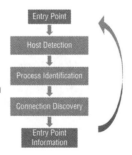

Figure 6.6: Service mapping process

From there the connection discovery begins by creating a host detection that is likely to result in a configurable CI. Then, the process ID starts to build out the requisite components that make up the service, and finally the connection discovery is completed by discovering what other connections exist to create the full mapping.

You can also do manual process mapping by looking at the patterns and finding similarities, as shown in Figure 6.7. You can search for patterns by looking at the application's signatures and identifying information, such as port used, which could help to map the service. For example, if you were using a web server and it was an Apache or Tomcat system, or by doing a file transfer and using the protocol FTP, you can find all of this information by looking for patterns. Although it goes way beyond the scope of this book, I wanted to make sure you at least knew it could be done because it needs to be done to have a complete system. Manual process mapping may be the reality in smaller enterprises that do not allow for scanning, discovery, and other intense probing. Manual process mapping may in itself cause a performance degradation of the operational systems.

NOTE   Manual process mapping is time-consuming. In fact, it can sometimes be out-of-date even before it is complete, leading to unreliable information.

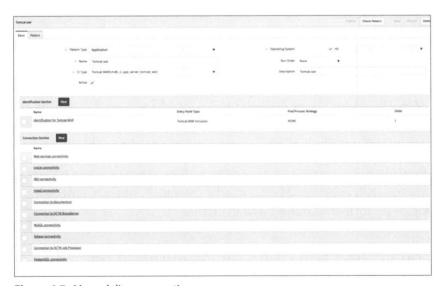

Figure 6.7: Manual discovery options

You can also design patterns and architected mappings based on connectivity. You can map via known items and find upstream and downstream dependencies that may need to be included in your service mapping. Here you can find configuration files, network connection information, and other metadata that can help to map dependencies.

Figure 6.8 shows the Pattern Designer, which you can use to design and build a map based on an application signature, other configuration items, dependencies, and connection information.

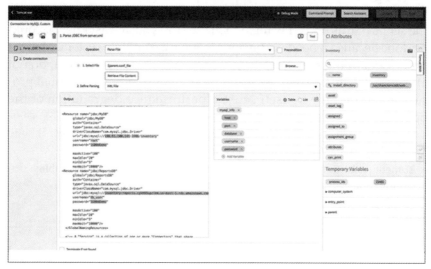

Figure 6.8: Pattern Designer

Once your services are designed and mapped and your AIOps platform is configured with automation and rules, you can test the system for accuracy. We can conclude that it is important to monitor and troubleshoot issues that occur with automation to ensure the best outcomes. Sending corrections to the AIOps platform will help machine learning functions improve their efforts and better handle situational issues. Consequently, AIOps performance output will increase.

Configuring and Using AIOps Automation

Once you have a CMDB that can be populated and an AIOps system that can use the information provided through mapped services, the next task would be to make sure that you configure AIOps to respond to event and fault management through automated actions. When working with a tool like ServiceNow, you can do all of this through the ITOM module. The ITOM will allow you to configure event management actions, and this translates to operational intelligence (OI). OI delivers analytical insight in a manner similar to AI.

Event management (EM) is the alerting, triggered alerts, alerts sent, captured, and created to signal a change on your baselined architecture. Alerts are triggered when events occur outside established baseline performance or limits, i.e., disk availability, network latency, and so on. Monitoring tools and other platforms to include in your AIOps system will all have a baseline of what is normal for an organization. You can configure these baselines yourself or allow the system to identify them through ML. ML has the ability to automatically set baseline parameters based on normal performance and can even adjust baselines for seasonal load changes. Once you have a CMDB and mapped services, you can configure actions based on changes. So, for example, you may have a database that needs to be indexed because you have a performance issue. You don't know that yet, but you will be told that by your AIOps system that is monitoring the baseline health of the service and its mappings. If the EMR is operating poorly and help desk tickets are being opened, you should already know that the database as part of that service is running at 98% CPU and causing a service impact. EM allows you to know this is happening because an alert should have been generated (and quite possibly a ticket) that alerts the responsible parties that a database is impacted and needs to be looked at.

Operational intelligence (OI) is the proactive response to issues (like AI) that allows you to prevent service outages using ML to predict or be proactive with what could happen based on known thresholds. For example, you might know that the CPU needs to be at 75% and can only spike higher for a few seconds or less. But if your CPU spikes and stays high for 3–4 minutes at or around 100%, then your service will be degraded. This should kick off an alert, but also an action to move the service to a responding system with a CPU that can handle it. Maybe the systems are load balanced, and one needs to be added to the pool to handle some of the load. Whatever the action, OI is responsible for taking action and helping you identify and proactively try to stop service outages from occurring or highly minimizing their impact.

NOTE   Remember, AI is not meant to replace people but to augment their effectiveness. It is all about allocating resources to get the best results possible for your organization and your clients.

Monitoring and Operating Event Management Services

Now the automation can take place and the true nature of configured AI, ML, and AIOps self-healing capabilities can be realized. In the next section, I will show you specifically how to use your AIOps platform to review your environment and how automation is set up, if AI and any other automated functions are working. In this example, I will use ServiceNow and the Operator Workspace, as shown in Figure 6.9. Here you can configure your EM environment in a way that allows you to view your mapped services and specifically their health and operation. You spent a lot of time and effort strategizing, designing, mapping, and building viable services in your AIOps platform; now it's time to realize their true potential. The Operator Workspace in ServiceNow can help you:

- Work with the mapped services, their displays, and what is represented and how. It filters specific services and controls the views of what you want or do not want to see.

- Group the services based on outage severity, service mapping groups, or other. This can help you to quickly see and review an outage taking place and what is affected. One of the key benefits of AIOps and specifically ServiceNow is that it groups alerts so the operator is not overwhelmed. This helps the operator quickly discover the root cause and remediate it. This will greatly reduce dependent alerts and help identify remaining ones that have not been corrected by handling the alert with the highest impact.

- View different alerts based on how they are mapped in the system and what the service mapping is showing, which is helpful so that you can quickly see if an alert is critical, what service or services it affects, and what it impacted.

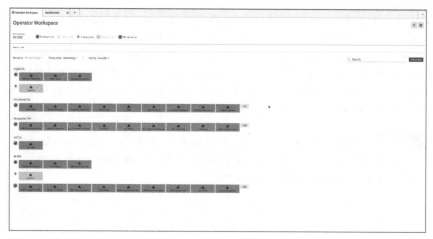

Figure 6.9: Using Operator Workspace

Note that Figure 6.9 shows the simple layout of the workspace to give you a snapshot in time. The Operator Workspace allows for an easy-to-understand and quick view of the status of critical services. For example, near the top of Figure 6.9, we have an order status marked as being in a critical state, which means that action needs to be taken quickly to restore the service. This is a customized view that shows the specifics of a service and its dependencies and how they are impacted by an issue. When you click the critical alert (Figure 6.10), the component (Order Status) is shown in critical state, and once selected, it will show you the top alert view, which points to a computer system and a fault that it has experienced. From here you can select the service details to learn more about it or select the service map to view the mapping of the service and all the impacted dependencies.

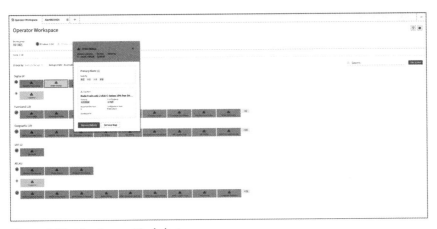

Figure 6.10: Viewing a critical alert

Once you select the map, you can see the alert in the bottom view and the affected Oracle server that is causing the outage or impact as seen in Figure 6.11. Color-coded items allow for a quick visual. What is most critical here is that an impacted database could create an impact for not only this service but many others that could be experiencing a similar outage.

As we drill down further and start to review the outage map, it's obvious that there is a disk space issue causing a disruption.

What is also clear, as shown in Figure 6.12, is that there are other dependencies as you look at other views of what the database impacts and how it's mapped. You can see there are web server frontends and multiple sources of middleware that could be experiencing issues, all from this disk issue. Figure 6.13 shows another view of the outage based on the mapping of the service.

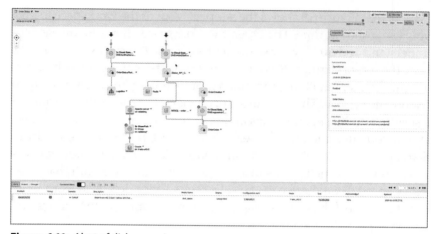

Figure 6.11: Alert of disk space issue

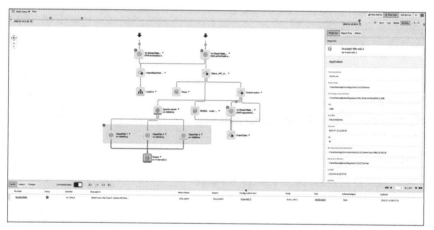

Figure 6.12: Viewing other dependencies

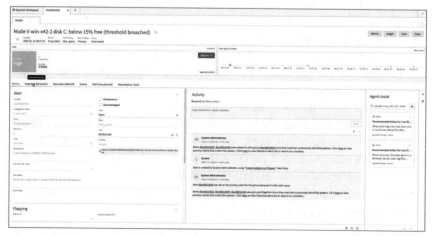

Figure 6.13: Viewing alert details and history

Once you select the alert, you can see that the threshold has been breached and why the alert was triggered in the first place. Here you can see that the severity is critical and that the impacted services are listed with an action and work notes. You can see a trail of other alerts that may have taken place (for example, if this is not the first time), the incident creation alerts, and any all other alerts that may have historically taken place.

This is the beginning of the AI function being based on historical data. The known history of outages and impacts is what root-cause analysis (RCA) data and corrective and preventative actions will help to identify. This is what can be used to start to build the automated and self-healing functions that are to come next.

This is where the fundamental basics of AI and ML start to take hold. Up until now, there has been a lot of data collection and analysis of that data. The event management platforms are able to collect a tremendous amount of data and show it to you, mapped out and in a way that helps you understand what you are looking at, but what happens when an event is triggered and the system is intelligent enough to know everything we just reviewed and discussed and make an educated guess on what the best cause of action is to be? In a clinical setting, this could be life or death. Failing over to another node would make the most sense. There are decades of design and strategy put in place within IT systems to create failover systems for this exact type of situation. A CPU node goes to 100% and is sustained. The system performance is degraded. The secondary node is online and waiting, and there is a failover event that takes place to restore service on a node that is at lower capacity and able to handle the requests or the load. The answers come from the past collected data. For example, in Figure 6.14, you can select alert insight and start to review what alerts have already taken place and what has been done to restore service. From here we can configure automatic handling of events based on what has been done before.

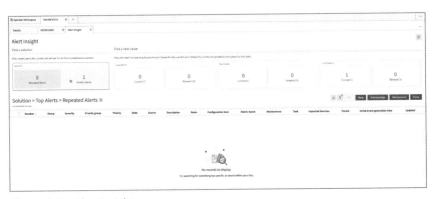

Figure 6.14: Alert Insight

By reviewing the past alerts and the actions that took place, there is hope that automatic handling of system events can be done by the AIOps platform (in this case with ServiceNow it would be ITOM), and AI could be realized as a trusted output to a failure, fault, or other event.

The biggest outcome (and what is to come next) is that now that you completely understand what has to happen based on your service mapping and over time what has taken place and occurred again, you are poised to see the true benefits of AI and ML in a way that both manual and automatic automation events can be created to resolve issues, cut tickets, restore service, and so much more.

> **NOTE**   Most of this book has prepared you for the realization that automation is the foundation of AI and ML when it comes to AIOps and most event management platforms. Years of research and real-life deployments have shown us that the truest form of machine learning comes from collected data and outcomes. Much like clinical research, you make wise decisions based on experience, and AIOps is no different. Now that you have spent a large portion of time strategizing, planning, and deploying an amazing system, it's creating the actions that will bring your ROI to the forefront of your capital investment.

Creating and Realizing Automation, ML, and AI

When all of the foundational items have been established and you have been running your system for enough time to capture data, your trusted data sources are configured and maintained, and all sources of information, like CIs and your CMDB, are updated and correct, you are ready to create and customize automated functions. This is where things get interesting.

When using a tool like ServiceNow, you can create automated functions in the Flow Designer, as shown in Figure 6.15. Here you can view, design, create, adjust, and analyze your automated functions. This is an example of a workflow that handles an alert and shows what you can do to enhance the process. Remember, this is the foundation for "automatic" handling of everything through AI and ML.

In the Flow Designer's dashboard, you can create new workflows, automated functions, and actions based on flows. Here you can see a new flow based on an incident process. For example, the subflow will be based on an incident (alert) that takes place and the actions needed for it to take place. In this instance, if the alert takes place and the device that is impacted is not in maintenance mode, then actions need to be taken.

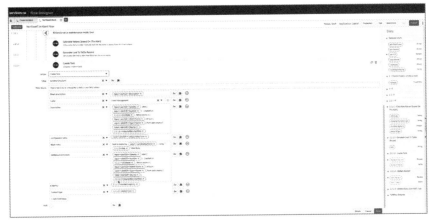

Figure 6.15: Using Flow Designer

Maintenance mode is when you place a system "off alert" so that you can do maintenance on it without triggering actions based on false positives. An example may be that you need to install a patch on a system and reboot it. If the system reboots (goes down and offline), it may trigger automation to take place. Therefore, it's important to place the system in automation mode so that you do not trigger the process of automation which may cause an issue. The other reason is that this could lead to tickets being cut automatically and sending the service desk into action by assigning engineers and so on. If there is no issue, there is no reason for such an effort. This is also something that happens often with change control via ITIL change management. When a ticket is open for change, the system normally goes into maintenance mode. As you can see, there are many factors that go into a simple single automated rule. This is why AI can be so tricky. With an AIOps system, each and every action has a reaction.

We can also see the Boolean math I spoke of earlier. In the example illustrated in Figure 6.15, the following items make up the entire flow:

- The flow is one function that contains subflow items. Each subflow item is based on the item before it. For example, IF the alert is not in maintenance mode, THEN do one of the next few steps.

- The next steps are also based on specific actions. Here we can see an example that says that IF the alert triggers and needs to be actioned, then the AIOps system needs to calculate severity and validate the CI information and urgency of handling and pushing to the next step.

▪ The subflow steps also point to creating a ticket (incident task), which may do one of quite a few things. For one, it can create a ticket and assign it to an engineer. In other instances, the tasks can be to run a script or run an application.

The Boolean IF, THEN, ELSE is the foundation of all the technology we will continue to develop with the workflow and process engineering, so make sure you continue to think through this flow of actions as you continue to develop more workflow.

TIP   You do not need to be a master of Boolean math (or any math) to become great at automation. As I have mentioned in the past chapters, having an understanding of the technology, functionality, designs, and how things work can take you far, and, in some instances, being a jack of all trades is okay in this situation. It is worthwhile to mention that the more you know about automation and what could happen, based on actions and reactions, the more you can help to design the intended actions. These are the building blocks for all AI and ML. AI and ML are heavily rooted in math, so you may want to start to learn more about it as you delve deeper into the subject in the future based on your role in the organization. If you are someone who is programming and working with automation, you may need to spend some quality time better understanding how the math works, which is not complicated but goes beyond the scope of this book and should be reviewed and learned as its own topic.

Figure 6.16 shows how you can further develop the actions you take or that will be taken. The drilling down into the flow can show more details on what actions to take next. For example, when we look at the handling of log files, there is more to review with the workflow. Here, IF the device is a Windows server (action 1), THEN you delete the logs, update the ticket, and so on. There is also an action 2 (and subactions) where IF the device is a Linux server , THEN you log, delete Linux log files, and so on.

What's important to take away from this lesson on automation is that your AIOps system will do the same thing based on manual or dynamic response. If your system continues to process this data (whether you configure it or it's configured by the system itself), you still need to understand it. It still needs to be reviewed, and it still needs to be tested, monitored, maintained, and updated. It drives home the concepts I started talking about in the first few chapters of this book that there are key takeaways to understand the value added by AIOPs, AI,

ML, and intelligently automated technology. There is no plug and play, especially on an enterprise system that is very large (or even small or medium, for that matter) or one that runs critical functions such as military, law enforcement, medical/healthcare, or other critical infrastructure where mistakes cannot be tolerated and can cost lives and large amounts of money.

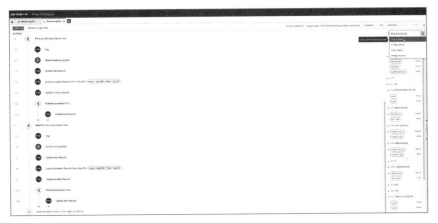

Figure 6.16: Creating automation

Automating Splunk and IT Service Analyzer

Taking a closer look at the automation of services, post-service mapping, and development, we can see the same framework used in another AIOps platform like Splunk. Although Splunk is as all-encompassing as ServiceNow and ITOM, there are many identical themes that you will find highly relevant to designing an AI and automation strategy.

Although the names are different, the operations usage is pretty much the same with a few differences that I will cover in this section. You can accomplish the same functionality with ITOM and Splunk using tools like IT operations modules and dashboards using the Splunk Artificial Intelligence for IT Operations solutions and its Data-to-Everything platform. It does this by collecting data, using it in a value-added way that will allow for insights and how to automate based on those insights. In Figure 6.17, you can see the Service Analyzer.

There is a need to map services so that there is an understanding of what you will automate. In this example, you can see that the Splunk Service Analyzer is one of the modules that you can use to identify what those service mappings look like when connected and ingested correctly and what automated functions you can create from them. It is similar to the ServiceNow solution. You can see that they are similar in form, as shown in Figure 6.18, where a simple tree view of the same data can show impact and how it drills down (or up) through your organization, the impacted service, other services that may connect to it, and so on.

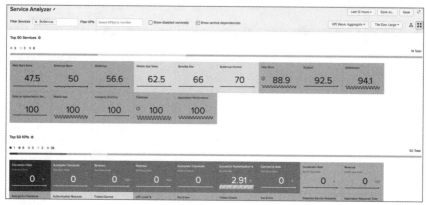

Figure 6.17: Splunk Service Analyzer

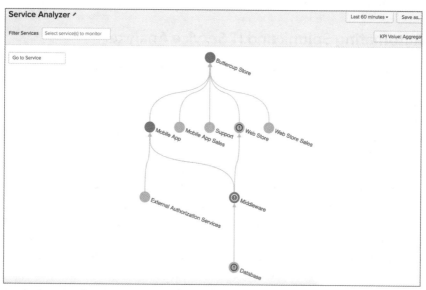

Figure 6.18: Splunk Service Analyzer tree view

When considering the Splunk Service Analyzer and its mapping component, consider the following:

- The process map is usually outlined with tree views representing a group or person who handles the task, process block, or decision that takes place. Each service component is laid out in a tree that allows quick viewing of impacted services.

- Each grouping shows a documented service based on CIs similar to ServiceNow. The similarity comes in that all ingested data into the platform starts to build maps that show dependencies that may in fact impact the service as a whole or portions of it.

- The service mapping may also show that one component, CI, or function could impact more than one configured service.

- The process itself is similar to a Boolean mathematical function. For example, IF a person does something specific, THEN a response will take place, or ELSE something different will occur.

- The process needs properly identified start and end points so that it is clear when adjustments need to be made to the process itself. You can compartmentalize process functions into subprocesses to improve maintenance and handling.

- You can make a process for practically anything you need to do. Learning how to lay out a process will be extremely helpful.

The concepts are based on AIOps where big data once snapped into a solution such as this (whatever platform you choose) remains the same. You need to remember the basics that were discussed earlier in this chapter's "Understanding Automation" section.

With Splunk, the tool will basically ingest data from sources, categorize the data, and then allow you to either manually or let the system dynamically work with that data in a way that allows it to automate actions. Do you need a CMDB? No. Other sources of data will suffice, but a CMDB is always preferred in any situation over others because it is usually considered the centralized data source of most master data management (MDM) program efforts in large enterprises. Health systems are normally the biggest users of data, and having an MDM is critical to successful analytics and informatics; however, in this use case, with IT operations and AIOps, it is similar in that this central source of data becomes the source for all. This is where the AIOps platforms do their analytics (predictive) to be able to automate actions based on events.

NOTE   Predictive analytics, the forecasting of possible events, fault management, event management, data analysis of source data, and conducting of statistical and metrical analysis are all the underlying components to a successful AIOps platform deployment and, more so, the configuration of designed automation to handle actionable events. Predictive analytics is what AI and ML need to actually handle automated events. The system looks at what has happened before, what is happening now, what thresholds are in place, and what automation is configured and makes action possible through prediction. This gives artificial intelligence its "intelligence," so to speak. The machine learns what to do based on historical data and predicts actions based on what it believes should take place to keep things in their operational thresholds.

Other basics of predictive analytics are anomaly detection and root-cause analysis review and corrective/preventative action handling. Anomaly detection is an important function that is nothing more than the triggering of events based on set or known thresholds. This has been an age-old solution used in most security products for decades. If something seems out of the norm, it's considered fishy and may be worth a look to ensure no issues are taking place. Similar to AIOps platforms, anomalies can mean problems. They do not always mean problems, however.

Earlier I mentioned Six Sigma and the processing of data, the review of it, its inputs and outputs, and whom the data serves and why. After running the DMAIC process, it's understood through statistical analysis tools and processing that you have a normal run of all processing and there are things that may not fit into that norm. These are called *outliers*. Outlier data includes things that you need to assess because they do not fit into the norm. When an AIOps solution processes data as normal and within a threshold, it needs to understand what is not within that range and specifically what to do if it isn't.

When looking at tools used in Six Sigma, such as statistical engineering tools to look at regression, distributions of collected data, and standard deviation, there is a method where you can create a dot plot, as shown in Figure 6.19, where data can be looked at on a plane.

This data when reviewed will show you what an outlier looks like within a normal threshold distribution. When you consider how a technology such as Splunk (or other platforms) better understands how to react to data and what actions to take, always remember outliers, and it will help you to better grasp how predictive analytics work based on anomaly detection. If a platform has specific known threshold markers, it's as simple as knowing that anything that steps outside the threshold (outlier) is an anomaly, it's detected (flagged) by the system, and some form of action is to be taken.

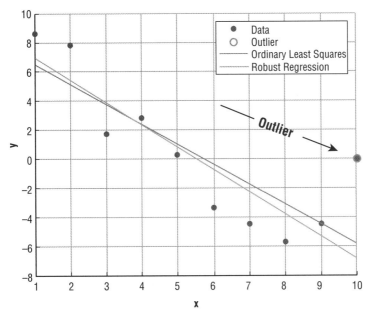

Figure 6.19: Analytics and outliers

Root-cause analysis (RCA) is another form of handling for detection and handling of incidents, events, and processing within an AI platform like Splunk or others. I covered RCA earlier in the book and spoke to its importance as it is one of the keys to having a stable ITIL service operations deployment in your enterprise. In clinical health operations, the ability to continue to provide healthcare is the goal of any IT operation behind it. IT ops is in place to keep that happening and the only way to do that is to keep systems stable and running. Problems will happen, and that is expected, no matter how hard we try to prevent them both proactively and reactively. That said, a good RCA program handled by a strong problem management (PM) process is going to provide you with the corrective and preventative actions necessary to keep a stable environment a reality. It is also the feeder for your AIOps platform because any "known" error is something that a threshold can be created on. A known error database (KEDB) can become a strong source of data to identify known outliers as they occur and the actions to take. Corrective actions may require something outside the scope of your AIOps platform, but preventative actions may be in scope. If a preventative action is to failover a system to a known good host, when an outlier occurs, that can be spotted by ML and handled by your automation, and stabilizing the system for clinical operations can become a reality.

Predictive IT is based on the ability to use a tool like Splunk, specifically the ITSI module (which is discussed in the next section).

There is a need to take all data like log files, up/down information, metrics, trusted sources, known errors, and more, and ingest them into a single source of analysis for intelligence to be derived from. We can look at that from the perspective of Splunk and its ITSI solution.

> **TIP**   Remember, the key to all this working is overcoming siloed data.
> Otherwise, your AIOps system may not have access to the logs and source
> data it needs to properly learn and predict possible issues.

Splunk IT Service Intelligence

Splunk uses a monitoring and analytics module called IT Service Intelligence (ITSI) to make AI and ML work. Everything discussed in the previous section regarding the sources of data, the mapping of services, and the collection of known issues and possible outliers based on threshold creates what is known as the Data-to-Everything platform. You can see an example of Splunk ITSI in Figure 6.20. Splunk ITSI using AI allows you to easily visualize your entire workflow with a single dashboard.

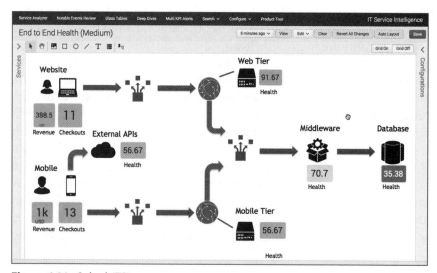

Figure 6.20: Splunk ITSI

As we look at the collected data and how it is portrayed in a dashboard, we can see relationships. When we try to better understand our environments in the form of services and service mappings, we want to know that we have what is called *end-to-end health*. This vision of what makes up end-to-end health is the culmination of all the configuration data and data sources such as how the service is used and how the information is collected. Once all of this is mapped correctly, decisions can be made on how to automate this data and how to do so manually or dynamically.

TIP   Application programming interfaces (APIs) are one of the key sources of ingestible data and something you should know about. An API is nothing more than a portal for your system to connect to and pull what it needs and/or be able to "interoperate" with another tool or source to get what it may need. An API is programmable and allows you to customize solutions. However, you may need a good programmer on staff to be able to handle advanced customizations. Simple connections and usage can be handled by most technical engineers you may have on staff today.

AIOps platforms and automation are making healthcare clinical outcomes better by improving efficiency, quality control, and better uptime for critical systems. Using a tool like ITSI will allow you to see your clinical operations and map it to your IT operations. ITSI will give you insights into how your service is operating and more. It can help you to automate actions that allow for continued uptime and use. If your EMR is mapped and in the AIOps system, any outlier can trigger an action. An outlier may be that your lab system is down and unable to provide lab functionality. This directly impacts your EMR. If your service analysis and mapping shows that a common database is down or it's impacting several services, you can view that impact in Service Analyzer and ITSI as well. This all creates better outcomes and allows for improved uptime, usability, and functionality. Remember, improving the user experience is the goal here, and when it comes to healthcare, it can mean life or death to keep usability and functionality at a high level.

Ultimately, automation is the functional arm of AI and ML that allows action to take place. Without automation, you have little more than a fault monitoring system.

HOW DO YOU KNOW IF AUTOMATION AND AI ARE RIGHT FOR YOU?

One of the marketing concepts for any AIOps platform is the selling of ROI. I have covered this topic a few times throughout the book because it's an important one and a recurring theme especially in the board room. You spend a lot of money on putting together, purchasing, and maintaining a platform of this size.

Consider these questions when getting ready to deploy your new system's automation capabilities and AI/ML functionality:

- Do you have a task that needs to be automated?

- Is it something that requires automation to be taken to the next level where automatic actions are taken based on the event that is triggered?

- Do you know what actions you want to take place?

- Do you know if there are alternate actions?

- What happens if the actions do not work or if they cause an issue?

- Do you know if automated actions can be trusted by a system to take action based on machine learning?

By knowing these answers, you are better positioned to know what you should or shouldn't deploy.

When Should You Use AI and ML?

A common question that comes up in executive circles and is answered by most if not all major AIOps platform developers is, should you use AI and ML? The entirety of this book has revolved around that question, and since the answer is highly complex, I have answered it in many ways throughout each chapter. The answer is complex, and that is why it must be re-asked and re-answered throughout the book.

How do you know if you should use AI and ML? Simple, you need to be connected to and understand the goals, objectives, and outcomes required for designing it correctly and deploying it smartly. Automation has been part of IT from the beginning with simple scripting languages all the way to the use of Ruby, Python, and many more commonly used and advanced technologies used today. Automation is not new. What is new is the discussion around it based on how it is used without tools that claim intelligence. Boolean IF, THEN, ELSE arguments have proven timeless and are the basis of triggering automation, helping ML to provide a better handling of alerts. Now, add in the tremendous amount of data and the analytics that help to create automated actions based on events that take place. Lastly, add in a system making decisions based on all of this data without your input (but not necessarily without your supervision; you still need to ensure that your systems are doing what you intend them to do). If you trust everything we have done so far, trust you know what you want to happen, and trust that you have a team monitoring and doing samples of outcomes in reporting and testing and it shows to be working, then the answer should be yes. You want the answer to be yes so you can get the ROI out of your investment. This book has aimed at making sure that you not only made the choice wisely, but also armed yourself with all of the work that needs to be done to make sure it's done wisely and continues to stay that way. Change causes disruption, and change is constant.

AI should be used if you are doing things that can be automated and trusted to happen without your knowledge but you still need to observe, monitor, pull metrics, review and report, and manage the system on a daily basis. This means you will have a footprint to manage even though many AIOps vendors explain that it reduces the footprint. It does if that footprint is large and doing redundant tasks that can be automated by a system that is configured correctly and smart enough to make those decisions. It must also be monitored, maintained, and updated accordingly.

One way to avoid a continued footprint (which I will cover in the next chapter) is using AI as a service or cloud operation, which can help augment staff. Smaller organizations find great value in this, but make no mistake, it comes with a cost, and you still need to manage and monitor the system at some level.

Summary

In this chapter, we took a look at AIOps technology and solutions from the perspective of task automation. This chapter discussed how healthcare systems can utilize their AIOps platform to reduce outages, improve service performance and availability, and improve overall system usage for clinical functions. Another aspect that we considered was automation and its importance in the AI and ML functionality. Whether you automate rules and actions via a manually created workflow or have the system build the workflow for you automatically based on learning what to do, it's the same process nonetheless. It's also important to understand how these things work because in critical environments you still need to monitor and maintain the automated actions based on what you expect to happen. This trains the ML to better avoid false positives, wrong actions, and inappropriate behaviors that cause more outages and setbacks to your deployment.

Once AIOps has been deployed and you are working with a fully operational tool, you can more successfully capitalize on the ways it can serve your organization. The ROI is improved by automated functions, and if you use any event management system like AIOps, you will see that to take full advantage of it you need to understand automated workflows. AI allows for the automated handling of workflows based on actions and reactions that the system encounters. Knowing Boolean math and understanding the concept of IF, THEN, ELSE can help to develop the needed information for machine learning and how to create functionality based on actions, flows, and subflows.

Although math needs to be understood, remember it is simply the foundation of how AI started. Boolean logic allows for the creation of automated actions called when machine learning is used to identify outliers and determines what actions should be taken or whether the alert should be assigned to an engineer rather than taking an automated action.

By setting up workflows, processes, and automation functionality within the toolset, you can begin to see how the AIOps system can really make an impact. Automation is the means that a system will use to create actions based on workflow setup and designed by process engineers. This chapter laid out the groundwork for how to review, process, and build a workflow that contains the anticipated outcomes you want to see. Once the system can learn, it can be used to create workflows based on use cases, scenarios, common outcomes, and more. To provide the best benefit, your system needs to be fully configured and include components like a CMDB, with trusted sources of data providing you with the foundational design for developing usable and trusted actions. In this chapter, we looked at all of the aspects associated with automation, workflow engineering, process engineering, and AI and ML. In the next chapter, we will explore the concepts of finalizing a project by deploying to the cloud and using most of these functions in an off-premise situation or hybrid, how that can impact your outcomes, and, most importantly, what security procedures need to be in place.

Cloud Operations and AIOps

"To penetrate and dissipate these clouds of darkness, the general mind must be strengthened by education."

—Thomas Jefferson

As you strategize and deploy AI operations (AIOps) into your healthcare setting, one of the most important considerations to take into account is where you will be hosting your platform. With today's move to cloud operations, many executives ask the same questions relating to hosting, and the number-one question is, "Should we move to the cloud?" The question may not be as easy to answer as you think. That is why the goal of this chapter is to demystify not only what is important about the cloud, but the reasons why you may or may not want to move some or all of your systems into a cloud hosting environment. I will explore all the pros and cons of using cloud systems, costs, challenges, preparation, deployment plans, migration, hybrid solutions, security of healthcare environments, privacy, and more.

This chapter discusses possible uses of the cloud in relation with deploying your AIOps system in a healthcare environment. Whether you deploy ServiceNow, Splunk, or any other form of AIOps system, you can rest assured that there will be a cloud hosting option available for consideration. Many people struggle with planning this correctly, especially with the complexity of the healthcare environment.

This chapter is about managing AIOps systems in the context of the cloud. I will explain what the cloud is and how its inner workings and underpinnings can work for you and not against you.

Understanding the Cloud

This section will explore what the cloud is, how it works, why you should consider it (or not), and the caveats, challenges, and benefits you may face moving forward with a cloud or hybrid solution. The cloud is not right for everyone. It is also incredibly difficult to get into the cloud when you have a preexisting noncloud environment to consider, especially in healthcare. The healthcare landscape also offers its own set of challenges primarily revolving around privacy, data protection, and legal guidelines an organization must follow. All of this will be covered so that you can make the best decisions for yourself, your company, your leadership, and those you service.

Understanding Cloud Computing

The *cloud* is simply a term used to describe a decades-old technology that has morphed over time into an on-demand service delivered by cloud providers. In cloud computing, customers lease or purchase services or other resources from a cloud provider over the Internet. Generally, for you as a purchaser and customer, the cloud is nothing more than a datacenter you connect to, lease space from, and host your services with. There are hundreds (if not thousands) of datacenters globally that are available to single users or entire companies over the public Internet.

There is much more to discuss and learn about, but we need to start from the beginning because it may be likely that you are working with traditional architecture in your healthcare system. The truth is, the cloud has been around for a pretty long time. It is a term that was coined years ago to basically say, "I have some extra space or capacity in my datacenter; if I sublease it to you for a price, you can use it." (This is similar to how people do commercial real estate.) Computer and IT companies jumped on the bandwagon immediately, turning a profit based on the expansion and rising costs of information technology. Because IT can be costly (and in fact is usually considered by the finance department as a cost center and not a profit center), CIOs, CEOs, and other senior leaders wondered how they could make money back on their investment. The answer was by using the cloud, which required an investment up front in expanded network infrastructure, storage networking, virtualized systems, and a high-level security architecture. It also required the investment in datacenter development where power, cooling, and other aspects of maintaining a high level of reliability and availability were critical to sustaining a model of 24/7/365 service. From there on, the cloud turned those who made that investment into managed service providers (MSPs) who offered the space, equipment, and professional IT technical expertise . . . for a price. The cloud was born, and it became the de facto standard for those who wanted to be able to leverage these services and also turn them off when they didn't need them. This is where elasticity comes in and why the cloud can be so valuable to so many.

Before we can fully understand today's cloud, we need to know how we got here. A brief tutorial will help you to better understand not only the cloud, but also virtualization, elasticity, and other key concepts you will need to grasp to navigate a cloud deployment. All this is important to know because many healthcare systems run old, antiquated, and mixed environments, which makes it complicated and, quite honestly, scary to go to the cloud.

Figure 7.1 shows the most basic network connectivity between two sites and depicts the most common use of a network, shared services, and access to resources from one site to another. It doesn't matter if the two sites are remote offices, datacenters, or a mixture of any type of site. The important thing is to know that there are resources accessed over a network that connects them both over a public or private network connection. In this example I have selected a private network connection that could be a T1, metro Ethernet, or other offered service from an ISP, MSP, or a telecom like ATT, or another provider.

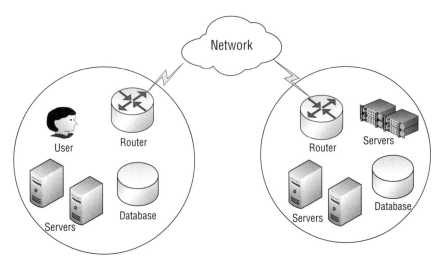

Figure 7.1: Traditional network connectivity

There are a few key factors that you must understand before considering what a cloud may encompass. For one thing, you have a user of some resources looking to access them over the network at their local site or a remote site, which the wide area network (WAN) connects them to. Looking at Figure 7.1, imagine a service of some kind hosted on servers located at the remote site. The following are key takeaways from this example:

- In Figure 7.1, there are two sites, but there can easily be more. I kept it simple for this diagram, but for this company where all resources are owned or leased by the company and kept "on premises," the ability to maintain privacy is held solely by those who work for the company, not a cloud provider. There could be multiple datacenters (for redundancy), multiple remote offices, and home satellite offices all connected to each other via a network.

- The network that connects all sites can be a private network or connected over the public Internet via virtual private network (VPN). Private and public network connections can both be encrypted, but when you use a public network connection, you stand more risk of interception, so using a VPN and encryption can reduce that risk.

- Every piece of equipment is owned, leased, and maintained by the company and the company's employees or outsourced vendors. All data is maintained by the company. All external access can be maintained from access to the company from external access points and monitored.

- Every component, technology resource, human resource, and other resources mentioned is a cost that must be maintained by both capital and operating budgets by the finance department; assets owned or leased must be amortized and maintained via asset management; and all contacts must be maintained separately by legal.

There are many more concepts to consider, but I wanted to point out some of the important ones since most healthcare systems today are either running in a traditional fashion or running as a mixture of old and new, which is called *hybrid* and is discussed later in the "Hybrid Cloud Solutions" section.

Figure 7.2 shows the layout of a site connected to the cloud. I collapsed the Internet connection into the managed service of the provider's datacenter to give you an impression of what the cloud is; however, it's nothing more than a different way of looking at Figure 7.1.

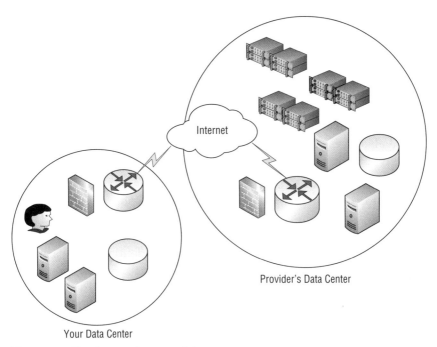

Your Data Center

Figure 7.2: Cloud network connectivity

It's a datacenter owned by another company that provides you with resources (storage, software, other resources) over a network connection. I want to be clear about the terminology and marketing verbiage used to create the illusion because that is all the cloud is: a technical sleight of hand that provides you with the same resources you could provide yourself, plus benefits. It's really all about your business model and the services and convenience you are willing to pay for. There are differences between hosting things yourself and having someone like a cloud provider host them for you. Some of the obvious differences include but are not limited to the following:

- **Connectivity:** Obviously, you connect to the cloud provider over an Internet connection, but everything behind it is transparent based on the level of service you are provided. I will get into the levels of service next, but the key here is that you connect to the cloud provider and get your service. It can be via the network connection itself, a portal, a remote access application (like Citrix), or something else. You can create connectivity to a datacenter, applications, or services directly from the Internet.

- **Ownership:** The off-premises hardware and resources all belong to the cloud provider, so you save a tremendous amount of money by not having to buy these things yourself. At the same time, you pay the cloud provider to host these things for you. So, you really need to do a cost-benefit analysis (CBA) prior to going to the cloud so that you know whether it's worth it. Giving up ownership removes the flexibility of having total control over everything, but it also frees you from the responsibility and costs of maintaining all of the hardware and other resources on-premises.

- **Security:** Security is probably one of the biggest concerns of any customer, especially those in healthcare. Keeping data private and confidential is not only the right thing to do, it's the law. There must be a level of security applied to a cloud-hosted environment that absolutely keeps all patient data confidential. There are concerns that a cloud environment may not be as secure, protected, or isolated as one may think and a breach could be extremely costly to the healthcare system hosting patient data on a third-party vendor's system. However, there are many HIPAA-compliant cloud hosting platforms. The important thing is to carefully research the vendor and determine its level of compliance and security.

- **Network connectivity:** Using the Internet is the preferred method for connecting in the cloud, although some cloud providers allow for private connections (which are generally more costly). The Internet, however, can be a challenge because it's not bandwidth you can always guarantee, and even though you are encrypting the data, it might be hacked in transit. The network connectivity should always be secure. This also increases the overhead (resource intensive) of the systems you are using. For example, if you access the cloud via a laptop computer over the Internet in order to access an application hosted on the cloud, the connection needs to be via a VPN and encrypted. This will create overhead, so your systems need to be able to handle this, which may require you to update older systems such as laptops, servers, routers, wireless access points, and other devices.

- **Service, resources, and allocation:** Resources can be elastic and somewhat limitless but costly. The one benefit to using a cloud provider is elasticity, which is something that many programmers, developers, and application designers love about the cloud. These environments can be created with virtual systems, storage, and networks. In place of the traditional hardware and decentralized model of the past, today's infrastructure relies on virtual servers (VMware being the biggest vendor in this arena) that can be "spun up" as needed. Even more importantly, the storage it uses can be added and sized based on what is needed. More CPU power? Add it. More memory? Add it. Don't need it? Spin it (or shut it) down. I can spin up a test environment, test or develop a system, and then shut it down afterward as soon as the test is completed. You pay for what you use, so if your payment or subscription model allows you to pay as you go, you can save money on spinning up and tearing down systems at will. This is not always the case when you own your own systems. You pay for them whether you use them or not.

■ **Management:** How your services and resources are managed is determined by your service offering (the various "as a service" offerings, which are discussed in the following sections). Staff may simply liaise with IT professionals who manage the systems, or you may manage them yourself based on contract. You may use a dashboard. You may have to provision services through a service ticket. You may need to escalate through the cloud provider's leadership or management for special handling or handling of issues. This requires you to liaise with the provider, so you need someone who knows how to work, open, close, and access service requests and handle service-related inquiries and issues.

TIP   A cost-benefit analysis (CBA) is what organizations do when trying to quantify the costs versus the benefits of doing something. When you consider going to the cloud, it sounds really enticing because the marketing around it makes it appear as though you won't have to own things, but it's really a displacement of money from capital purchases to an operating budget. You don't have to maintain equipment, bills, agreements, relationships, and health benefits for additional staffing, but make no mistake, you pay for them through the cloud provider who needs to do these things. Make sure that you completely understand the CBA of moving to the cloud as you may find giving up your flexibility of ownership may not be worth the 2% overhead in savings you projected by going to the cloud. The cloud should be something you move to for many reasons, not just cost savings.

> **TIP**   Keeping data private and patient data confidential is a priority of
> all healthcare systems. With tools and applications, it's easy for audits to be
> performed (or alerting) if someone who is unauthorized is looking where
> they shouldn't. Whether you keep systems internally or apply them to a cloud
> environment, tools can be used to audit unauthorized access of data and
> breaches.

In the next section, I will discuss the different "as a service" offerings
so you are aware of what is important when it comes to selecting options
within a cloud provider.

Cloud as a Service

When you think of the cloud, you think of a service provider. A cloud
service provider has a menu of sorts, and this menu provides you with a
variety of options to suit your needs. So, what does "as a service" mean,
and how do you select from a seemingly endless list of service offerings?
Originally when cloud first became a thing, it was simple and primarily
comprised three basic offerings. You had software as a service (SaaS),
platform as a service (PaaS), and infrastructure as a service (IaaS).

The common characteristic of the SaaS, PaaS, and IaaS offerings is
that they each follow the same model I had highlighted in Figure 7.2.
The main difference between the three of them is the span of what is
offered. Here is a breakdown of the basic service offerings and their
main differences:

- **SaaS:** Traditional SaaS offerings normally provide access to an
  application (or service) through a login provided by the cloud
  provider. Some of the first and oldest in this arena were finance,
  HR, and customer relationship management (CRM) tools that were
  too costly for smaller companies to own but were needed to handle
  their business requests. A common one that was used was
  Salesforce.com for CRM, sales, and marketing services. The most
  common application of use would be to sign up, pay a monthly/
  yearly fee, and be given credentials to a portal where you could
  access a shared system used by all clients.

- **PaaS:** Similar to SaaS, you will be given the same type of access
  to your systems. However, you are given more access to systems
  you pay for. What this means is if you were using a CRM tool, you
  may be able to access the application itself and control user settings, handle configuration settings, manage the APIs, write and

deploy code with the applications, control add-ons, and do much more. This is normally where you step into the role of development and need to access the system itself to test and deploy code.

- **IaaS:** IaaS can be considered the most expansive of the other offerings. Like the other two, you still need to connect to and access your systems in the cloud; however, you have access to more of the underlying infrastructure such as routers, switches, firewalls, and storage devices that are hosted within the environment.

With the advent of these three service offerings, most were pleased with the flexibility they provided. You could either pay less and have less control or pay more and basically manage an entire datacenter off-premise based on your needs and comfort level. Many leaders decided between the year 2000 and now to start (or continue) to move their datacenter operations outside the walls of their brick-and-mortar locations not only because of the cost but because of the need to keep their services running in case of a disaster. This wasn't an all-or-nothing proposal either. Some companies chose to keep some applications and data in-house and others in external datacenters based on their business needs and goals.

For example, in New York City after 9/11, there was a mass exodus of locally hosted datacenters to move them to a managed service provider or cloud provider because of the fear that any company that did not have a secondary datacenter could lose everything immediately if another disaster happened. The outsourced datacenters could provide a level of redundancy that in-house solutions could not provide. Certain functions (like CRM and legal) were outsourced to cloud providers that could host the applications they needed from a safe location. At present, more companies have managed to get through the initial shock of that tragic day and have been steadily deploying what is needed within the walls of the company and outsourcing the things not needed to hosting providers such as cloud management companies. The truth is, it really takes serious analysis (think CBA) to come up with the right solution for you. An example could be if you were setting up a monitoring solution for your healthcare system, you could consider running a test in a cloud environment like Amazon AWS first; then, once the proof of concept for your pilot is proven, you could choose to host internally or externally. Some offerings, like ServiceNow, are only cloud-based, so making a decision like that can be easier if you want to use that platform. However, if you choose to use other offerings, like Splunk that could be hosted internally or externally, then portions of your platform could be internal, while other portions (or even a backup platform) could be external. There are many ways to deploy your platform, as we will see in the upcoming sections on deploying and configuring AIOps in the cloud.

> **TIP**   You will need to understand the service offerings to plan for your AIOps platform in a way that allows you to communicate with the vendors wisely so that you can design and deploy an operations platform that delivers on your initial investment. I talked about ROI in previous chapters because it's an important consideration when it comes to purchasing AIOps and integrating it into your environment. You need to know what your options are and what the costs could or may be. Knowing cloud options allows you to make the best decision for what is right for your company and what is cost effective for the initial deployment and ongoing costs to maintain the system.

Now that you know the basic three models of cloud service, there is a fourth that is a more recent option. Functions as a service (FaaS) is a cloud computing category that is a step below PaaS where instead of spinning up virtual machines (VMs) and other application programming systems, you can spin up a function to test an application or service.

The cloud "as a service" options have expanded over the years to include many different well-known or not so well-known services, such as blockchain as a service (BaaS), database as a service (DBaaS), and mobility as a service (MaaS). In all honesty, it has gotten to a point where there are literally dozens of "as a service" offerings you can find online. Regardless, our current focus will be on the ones that matter to us: AI, ML, and AIOps, all of which are cloud functional services and come in "as a service" offerings. AIOps as a service is not technically a name; however, you can get an entire cloud functional AIOps platform. Artificial intelligence as a service (AIaaS) and machine learning as a service (MLaaS), however, do exist in technical terms and publications.

AIaaS is highly marketed via the Splunk platform sales and marketing team as an ML data platform that provides continuous insight into your enterprise via their AIOps platform. Splunk is an option that provides in the cloud a service analyzer, dashboards, and other logic tools to be able to conduct event and fault management, workflows and automation, and other configurations much as if you had it running on your internal network. ServiceNow (SN) with the ITOM module is also cloud-enabled and allows for AIaaS.

Other platforms, such as Dynatrace, Solarwinds, Cisco/AppDynamics, CA/Broadcom technologies, Riverbed, Oracle, IBM, and Microsoft, all follow suit. AIOps leaders have cloud solutions that help to enable a deployment, migration, or hybrid mix for whatever your needs may be.

Hybrid Cloud Solutions

Hybrid cloud solutions allow you to implement cloud solutions with traditional solutions. In a cloud-centric landscape, it's easy to get caught up in a cloud service provider's offerings, promises, and marketing pitches. What you need to do before you make any decisions, sign any contracts, or commit any monetary assets is to go back through the first few chapters of this book and make sure you did your homework on what you need to do with your AIOps platform and how it may work with your current infrastructure. What you will find is that most companies move to the cloud slowly, cautiously, and specifically. With a SaaS solution, it's easy to do because you outsource an entire app and its functionality and allow the company to manage the backend computing while you and your staff handle the front end. For some applications that works very well and can produce positive ROI. In some instances, it's cheaper to keep the solution in-house and manage it locally. There may be times when you decide to move your company to a new datacenter and the cost of redeploying is too costly; therefore, moving a portion of your service to the cloud makes sense. There are times where you do in-house development of services, software, apps, or other functions and doing a portion of it in Amazon Web Services (AWS) makes sense. This is where you want to be in the planning stages of deploying an AIOps platform in your healthcare environment. You want to know what the strategy is prior to doing so and make sure you do it in a way that makes sense.

There may be problems with deploying a solution because you may be connected to other sites such as partners. Similarly, if you have done mergers and acquisitions (M&A), you might not have completely brought in a company where you manage their IT systems. It may be that you plan to do so when these systems age out and are in need of updating or replacing. At that time, you may decide it's cost effective to connect them completely to your network and standardize their equipment. M&A scenarios may also result in a situation where you have hospitals running on one EMR or a Revenue Cycle system that is not up to the standard of what the corporate company is using. It would cost millions to convert the system. Nevertheless, there are conversion systems in place, integration tools, and other functions to get everything to work together. However, an AIOps platform may not be able to manage the same way across the board. Because of all of these challenges, many companies move to a hybrid approach when going to the cloud.

Figure 7.3 shows the basics of a hybrid cloud connectivity diagram. Here you can see everything I talked about when considering the bigger picture of having resources on your local network that you access over your network and other resources you may access from the cloud provider over a secure VPN-encrypted connection via the Internet.

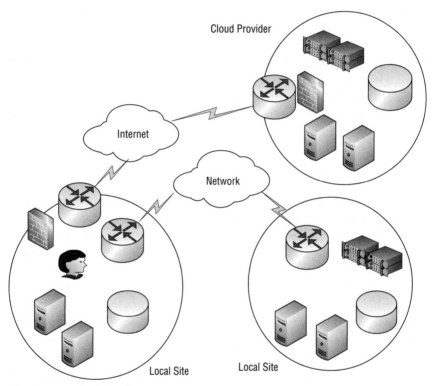

Figure 7.3: Hybrid cloud connectivity

Note that Figure 7.3 is the fundamental layout of what this may look like, and it can expand to multiple sites when we have multiple cloud providers delivering services. The hybrid cloud is nothing more than the use of both your private network and the cloud provider's systems in a managed remotely hosted datacenter accessed over the Internet.

TIP   Remember your terminology when it comes to dealing with cloud providers. The cloud is nothing more than a datacenter managed by a company where you pay a fee to lease their assets usually on a contractual basis. A hybrid cloud allows you to use your personal and private network along with this remote datacenter. A colocation is another term for the use of a rented datacenter where you store systems that you manage or co-manage with the provider. The colocation offers everything a traditional datacenter would but for a fee, of course. One of the advantages of co-location is that you have round-the-clock network engineers monitoring your server. This is similar to a cloud provider's IaaS offering. You'll also want to make sure that all cloud providers, colocation datacenters, and aspects of your system are HIPAA-compliant.

A hybrid cloud is great for healthcare systems that are looking to get into the cloud but have not been able to make the full jump inside. A hybrid allows you to convert systems slowly, test them for functionality, and make sure that you do not disrupt the providers, clinicians, and most importantly the patients who rely on these services.

WARNING   One of the most important design elements of going to the cloud is the use of the public Internet. This is especially true if you are running a critical cloud-hosted service that you and your clients (patients, clinical staff) can be cut off from if the network goes down. Reliability is important when deploying any service, especially one that could result in outages that cause disruption or mistakes that could lead to accident or death. Because of this, it's important to consider the design of your network and make sure that you have redundancy and resiliency baked into your design. This comes in the forms of disaster recovery planning (DRP) or business continuity planning (BCP) options in your deployment.

Hybrid clouds also offer the most flexibility when it comes to further expanding or decreasing your cloud footprint. If you have a cloud presence as well as an internally hosted and owned datacenter, you can make decisions quickly that allow you to pull back from the cloud if you need to.

Whether using cloud or hybrid cloud solutions, security must also be considered as well as compliance, regulations, and risk. When planning the scope of preparing an AIOps platform for use with the cloud, you need to make sure that you are considering security and that your cloud provider is too. Periodic audits of the vendor and their security by a team of in-house security experts or external consultants should be considered to test and make sure that your systems (and your data) are in fact secure and remain that way.

When You Should (and Shouldn't) Consider the Cloud

This chapter has discussed many of the aspects of the cloud. However, you should know what the pros and cons are of a cloud deployment so that you can more carefully consider your options.

Cloud computing is a mature solution. In the past, fewer people were excited about going to the cloud because they were nervous about putting their reputation (and careers) on the line if the cloud deployment went badly. It's a big cost up front. You sign contracts. You move critical data, resources, and assets to another location that you do not own. Lack of ownership is a big concern for those who move to the cloud. It's your data, but it's running on someone else's systems, in someone else's datacenter. One of the ROI concerns for moving to the cloud and going to an AIOps solution is reducing the footprint in both the managed system and staff, which should lessen the burden on your IT budget. By transferring ownership, you put it on the cloud provider (for a large cost) to handle (but for a cost, of course). That can be seen as a benefit. However, when you have a system go down and you get less of a response to resolve it from external teams than your own, the impact may be so severe that your immediate response is regret for doing this migration.

I have seen this first hand with priority systems such as enterprise resources planning (ERP) systems that, once hosted off-premise, didn't get the same quick response to issues that the internal teams could handle themselves. In healthcare where seconds could mean life or death, many people have a hard time with this lack of ownership and the ability to respond quickly to system outages on externally hosted systems.

Security is also another major concern. Knowing that their own staff may (and may not in some cases) be more trustworthy or committed to the company and its privacy, security, and trade secrets keep many from hosting systems externally.

Benefits include the use of large-scale computing power and the use of a greater amount of resources that could not be afforded otherwise. For example, if you were to do an exercise on big data (like you may for an AIOps platform), the large-scale storage platforms via the hosted SANs and the high-level computing power they offer can be a huge benefit when leveraged correctly. Advantages of cloud computing are also important when hospitals have many locations operating and the cloud solution helps AIOps integrate all of the data.

The biggest benefit is elasticity of resources and the ability to spin up and spin down instances of anything allowing you the time to test, develop, or use systems and computing power on an "on-demand" system. This allows you to pay for what you use when you use it. It also allows you to shrink the footprint of storage, virtualized systems, network, or access control whenever you need. A smaller footprint (locations, power, bills, electric, network, humans) allows you to reduce the need to manage all of these items separately, which is another benefit to elasticity; however, it does all come with a cost and, again, a lack of total ownership and control.

NOTE   In some instances, some of the top solutions are only cloud-based or are highly recommended for use in the cloud.

Challenges of the cloud are not many, but they can be significant depending on what your needs are. A hybrid allows you to toe the line. It's not an all-in solution; however, you want to make sure that you don't stay out in situations where it is obvious you can go in. Make sure you make good decisions. However, the challenges of AIOps and healthcare solutions in the cloud can be even more serious if you hover in between and incur costs for both with limited ROI. Often, after testing and analyzing your options, the benefits of moving in one direction or the other seem obvious.

Deploying to the Cloud

Now that you have a great background on cloud providers, cloud computing, what works, and what doesn't, you can start your deployment to the cloud based on this knowledge. A lot of the information I provided in the first few chapters of this book can help you plan a deployment correctly, especially to the cloud. Much of what I covered already can help you with the preliminary scoping of the project, how to manage the project correctly, and how to get it accomplished. I will not repeat all of that because it's basically the same information. However, I will discuss differences and caveats.

One of the biggest challenges in deploying to the cloud is whether to pick a cloud, noncloud, or mixture (hybrid) of the two. What makes this decision more difficult is the use of preexisting systems in your environment.

Figure 7.4 depicts a situation where an internal source of data and its servers are an enterprise's current event and fault monitoring and management solution. The data needs to stay intact while preparing and then executing the deployment of a cloud-hosted version, as shown in

Figure 7.4. There are many things to consider in this scenario. For one, when working in any type of critical service environment such as healthcare, you need to consider keeping systems functional during deployments. If you are to have a controlled outage via change management, you need to have a plan for receiving alerts and know when systems are impacted when migrating or deploying a new AIOps platform.

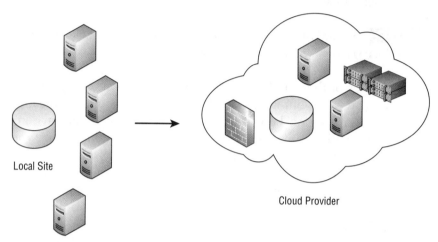

Local Site

Cloud Provider

Figure 7.4: Migrating data from a local source to the cloud

Here are some of the challenges:

- **Security:** Security is always a concern when you are connecting from a private secure network to a vendor's network to host data or have those systems check and monitor your internal systems. That means you will need to consult with security specialists to ensure that you are doing everything they expect you to do regarding following firewall rules, logging, audits, intrusion detection, encryption, and risk assessments as well as scanning, vulnerability testing, penetration testing, and other important security functions to keep your network, applications, and data secure.

- **Networks:** Connecting to another network means that you need to probably do some form of network address translation (NAT), set up and configure routing, and understand the network hops, which may add latency, or what bandwidth is needed to avoid putting too much pressure on your Internet connection. All of this needs to be assessed and tested for performance so that you know the solution works, but you are not impacting other applications, systems, or functions that use the Internet connection. This may also put pressure on the protected network segment usually called the *demilitarized zone* (DMZ), the network firewalls, and other equipment that processes data in the form of packets from one network to another. Monitoring is constant, so it may put a lot of pressure on your protected segment.

■ **Performance:** VPN/encryption equals slow performance, so all of the overhead I just mentioned with security and networks, including all the devices, servers, and systems where CPU, memory, disk, and other resources reside, may take a performance hit. When encryption is used it adds the need for more resources, which may impact the resources available for these other services when VPNs are used.

■ **System syncing and updates:** These may also put pressure on the network and the Internet connection. If you have systems that are going online or offline or are adding, moving, changing, syncing, or replicating data, especially from database to database, all of this can impact the connections and create performance loss.

■ **Using both systems:** Dual-purpose systems can simultaneously put an unwanted burden on host computers as well. This applies to all of the other items in this list. If both are running at the same time, it will create a possibility where you have twice the resource burden. One potential example of a dual-purpose system would be a server running both a database and a web server.

■ **Possibility for errors:** Errors can happen while deploying or when things are missed during normal operations. Errors can take place because of the added complexity of the migration or deployment.

Although this list is not exhaustive, it is enough to get you thinking about the myriad of issues that can take place during deployment. It is also not meant to scare you, but to alert you to the many facets of deployment. Deploying an AIOps system is a big undertaking and requires a massive deployment plan that is well thought out and completely assessed from start to finish for any problems, mistakes, or issues. It's a tall order, but it's one that needs to be attempted to ensure that not only are clinical staff not impacted, but there is no loss of system management that keeps everything operational including the EMR, revenue cycles systems, and other key and critical systems for the healthcare system. If all of these details are followed, you will be in a great position for a successful deployment. This is also the reason that companies recommend incremental deployments of AIOps rather than trying to deploy every system simultaneously.

NOTE   One of the ways to work with a preexisting vendor (or a new one) is to ask for a proposal. The official business term for this is a request for proposal (RFP). This way you can leverage your buying power and brand. If you are a large healthcare provider or system, there is value in your brand. Asking multiple vendors to come to the table and seek your business should be as simple as asking their sales team for an RFP.

Conducting a Request for Proposal

Conducting a request for proposal (RFP) process can really help you establish a budget up front for your AIOps deployment. Often, a good RFP process can help you develop your project plan, scope, and deployment process. An RFP may come from the vendor your organization already works with (such as your current tool vendor) or their competition. You can research top vendors by running a simple Google search on AIOps, which will pull about a dozen pages of vendors you can look at and contact.

The RFP process can also be modeled by your organization to identify what you want the vendor's proposal to address. For example, you want the vendor to understand what your goals are with the deployment. You want them to know what concerns you may have up front so they can answer them. You may want to clearly state your objectives, goals, scope, and expectations so they can answer them in clear language. You may want to ask them how they can do the work better than their competition, what makes them different, and how they plan to create a great product with a flawless design and deployment plan.

You will also want to know how they add value to the product with their team. You will definitely want to know what their support model is for their product. For example, if they are a newer company, have they regression-tested their system on big clients? I have seen this in the past where smaller companies look to hook the big fish so they can use them in their sales and marketing data. For example, I would ask a company what other companies similar to mine they have serviced successfully, who they were, and whether I can get a reference. A company like ServiceNow has hundreds of customers at the highest level, so their RFP will likely contain this information but with this comes a higher cost. A smaller company looking to gain a foothold may come in at a considerably lower price; however, they may not have the ability to correctly service a company your size and with your complexity. All of this can be worked out through the RFP process, and I highly recommend you take this step with an AIOps deployment especially for a critical service like a healthcare system.

You should consider a few more things regarding the RFP process. The vendor and sales team should come to the table with solutions to your problems and be able to answer all your questions or come back with answers if they cannot answer them directly. They should be fair and realistic and so should you. These companies are looking for a sale, and you are looking for a product and service. So, you are both looking for mutual gain and advantage. Although you may be defensive and on guard, most companies do not want to screw up a deployment to a client because it's in their best interest to not only make you a happy client, but to also get a good reference from you for future work. Your success is their success and a steady income on payments made for service.

Your goal is to receive what you need based on what you outlined and have the vendor provide you with what you expect. There may be times when you are unsure of what is needed, or you are certain you know but after the design discussion, the scope may change based on learning about new options. A good knowledge about the products, vendors, services, and uses of the tools you are considering helps you in making a purchase. You can meet in the middle successfully by knowing what the options are, what you want to set as a project scope and objective, and what the combined team(s) can achieve together. The RFP would also set rules and boundaries for cloud-hosted solutions where you may need to pay a renewal fee, monthly or annual fees, or other fees associated with the service. It would behoove you to take the time to scrutinize all aspects of the RFP, and the contracts, and even have the legal team involved before signing anything. You need to know what your options are if you stay with a cloud vendor, or, in some instances, if you need to back out of the solution.

TIP   Although it may cost you, you may be able to work out pricing for deployment assistance. In many organizations, this is worked into the cost and sale of the system where consulting hours are designated to assist with the deployment to help navigate many (and ideally all) of the issues you may come across while deploying to the cloud. Although this is extremely helpful, it does add to the costs of the deployment and is usually appended to the operations budget. A pro tip is when selecting a vendor and having them do a presentation to win your business over other vendors, work out a plan to get training and deployment costs lowered during the initial cost assessments.

Additional Deployment Options

There are other options besides replacing (also known as *forklifting*) or deploying a new AIOps system. There are upgrade options and integration options as well. Another option is if you have the base platform deployed and are adding AIOps functionality to it. You do not always need to rebuild from scratch, and sometimes, this is not only out of the scope of your budget allowance, but also highly impactful to the entire organization. Within healthcare systems there is a goal to have system availability at an all-time high and reduce impact as much as possible to keep clinicians doing what they do best. There may be a solution where your current monitoring and service desk platform can be upgraded to a newer more robust version where AI and ML can be leveraged. Most of the vendors are looking into AI options and either have deployed them or they are on the product roadmap.

For example, you may have a system deployed, and it may offer a new module (upgrade) that allows you to have AI functionality. For example, Computer Associates (CA), now merged and owned by Broadcom, has older CA Service Desk systems that are now being upgraded with AIOps functionality. The entire service line has been upgraded and brought into a futuristic version of new artificial intelligence solutions. By upgrading your current systems, you can move to AIOps within your current platform, which will enable you to keep your current business relationships intact and perhaps get better purchasing power for your budget. It reduces the impact, downtime, and burden of your organization. Sometimes it makes sense to build on what you already have before you consider pulling everything out and rebuilding from scratch. Figure 7.5 shows an example of a new platform version of an AI solution from an older platform.

Most systems today offer the same grouping of services and are based on large data sets that are collected and analyzed. This is the main reason I focused so much on big data and the practices used to analyze it in Chapter 6. You will see that as we move into the future of AI and ML (Chapter 8), the data sets will become even larger, more integrated, and with distributed computing power sources to crunch, manipulate, and analyze data even more closely to make automated (AI/ML) decisions that are more on target than ever before.

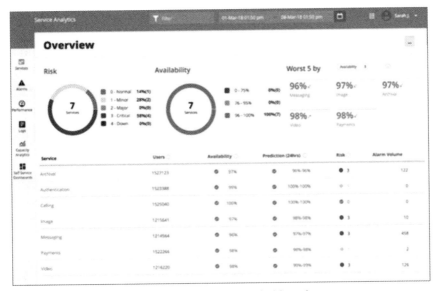

Figure 7.5: CA/Broadcom AIOps Service Analytics dashboard

Another option (and probably the most complicated one) is a system of systems. Anyone who has worked in IT long enough has experienced the interconnection of dissimilar systems by "getting them to work together" at some point. If you have not and are unaware, then I can assure you it's an IT professional's least favorite thing to do. Today, it's less costly, easier to manage, and easier to forklift or deploy new than it is to figure out a way to get things to work together, but alas, there will be times when the business needs and mission dictate the necessity of taking this course of action.

Normally, good design practices will immediately make you shy away from ever doing this, but there are business situations that create this design out of many factors. These factors include but are not limited to the following:

- **Mergers and acquisitions (M&A):** There will be times when your organization looks to grow by merging with, partnering with, or outright buying other companies. In healthcare, this may come in the form of buying other healthcare IT (HIT) companies, hospitals, practices, or other companies like insurance groups. When this happens, the connection of the two may be large, and replacing everything at once would be prohibitively expensive. You may have a plan to replace things in the future, but for now you must use what you have. Because of this, you may be forced to find a way to make both systems work together. For example, if you have two sets of monitoring systems, they have to be used in tandem.

▪ **Cost:** As I just mentioned, there may be a need to wait until there are funds available to grow your current platform with the new acquisitions or connections.

▪ **Use:** Use of and disruption from migration can cause clinical disruption, which may require you to keep things in place while creating a new platform that will be used in the future. Slow versus fast deployments or migrations can cause you to have two systems in use at the same time while you are migrating.

▪ **Necessity:** Some systems might be unique in providing essential functions that are not offered in other systems. Other times, systems have been customized where they are needed, and disruption is not an option.

Every one of these use cases can cause you to have a system of systems that involves keeping multiple systems online at the same time. This system of systems sometimes includes multiple dissimilar systems in use while maintaining operations by merging various separate groups, some of which have AI systems and others of which do not. It is important that you plan, scope, and choose solutions that allow you to integrate such a system of systems effectively. You can accomplish this by employing the techniques discussed throughout this book thus far and incorporating all relevant stakeholders while doing your research.

Once you have deployed your systems into the cloud, our last step is figuring out the basics of managing them. This won't be a long section because it will be similar to what you have already learned in the past few chapters except that access may be different. What is different and what I want to focus on is how you migrate into the cloud with your current IT staff and how that changes things for you and for them.

Managing in the Cloud

Managing your AIOps platform in the cloud should be as seamless as if you were working from your own internal system or over your cloud-hosted systems. One of the biggest differences is the network and where you may be accessing the cloud from. For example, you may have all of your systems managed under your Splunk instance that is hosted over a cloud. You may have all of your systems connecting and reporting to ServiceNow ITOM via the cloud. You need to manage those systems in the cloud from your current location whether it be within the walls of your organization or your home office where you may be working from. You may be at a hospital in the meeting and need to check something. Regardless of each situation I mentioned, you need to know what that means in regard to the management of these systems and how they connect to your AIOps platform and management of the AIOps system itself.

IT staff may also be using new processes and workflows due to the transition to the cloud. For example, you may have previously had a large contingent of IT workers managing the systems inside your organization and now you rely on the cloud provider to do that. You may need to retain these team members for new roles in the organization. Some of the new roles are critical to your success as a business operating from the cloud.

For example, some of your IT staff can fill the role of business relationship managers (BRMs). BRMs between your company and the vendor would be engaged in working out the details between your company and the vendor. BRMs need an IT background to be able to discuss things like service outages, metrics, reporting, business needs, IT needs, and how clinicians work with the systems in the cloud. Sometimes, this role can be shared where an expert in business is matched up to an expert in technology to deliver a full service to a client.

Service lines are also critical within healthcare environments. Unless they work in healthcare, most people do not know that a healthcare system is actually quite large, complicated, and multifaceted. The electronic medical record (EMR) is only one aspect of technology in a healthcare company. There are many others such as billing, revenue, scheduling, labs, and telemedicine, just to name a few. All of these require service lines of experts who know how to bridge the technology to the clinicians who use them. This is no different when you think of AIOps in the cloud and, quite frankly, just as large and complex. You are enabling all of your technology systems to be event monitored and automated through a cloud provider. So, you need to bridge the service line to the BRM or technology experts and then to the cloud provider to offer a full line of service between the business needs, how they map to the technology requirements, and what the cloud provider can offer as a service.

How AIOps can be used with the cloud is simple. You can manage your platform the same way you would without the cloud. The differences are in access and performance. The main forms of access may be a web browser, an application, a dashboard link, a mobile app, or through a console. Each form of access brings about a need for security over the Internet into the cloud provider's platform, and based on the "as a service" offering you selected, you may have other differences in how you manage and monitor the systems you are using. If you are using a SaaS solution, it's unlikely you will need to manage the servers that the application sits on; however, understanding what your SaaS solution does and how it works is important for the BRM. This way, if there are outages, performance problems, or other issues, the BRM can articulate it correctly with the cloud provider service team to get it rectified. It's important that the BRM be part of the AIOps solution.

Other issues that may occur are with performance. Performance degradation is a common, constant, and continuous problem for anyone who works with IT systems. Performance degradation is common because any time companies grow, usage grows, needs continue to grow, and the overhead used by these systems grows as well. For example, you may have correctly sized the bandwidth needed for your enterprise to service its current operations. However, placing the overhead of a management tool over the Internet to the cloud provider may cause an unforeseen bandwidth restriction or contention problem.

The encryption used may put an added burden on the resources of devices that service your enterprise. If the healthcare system is running a large amount of business over the Internet and you place a new AIOps system in the cloud and have 2,000+ machines reporting back and forth, this may result in resource usage surpassing current thresholds (at very high levels), causing performance problems.

Mobile users will definitely be a challenge for privacy, security, and performance. Also, compatibility may become an issue. Every cloud provider is going to tell you that you can access them via the web or a mobile device. Every AIOps vendor either has or is developing an app so you can access their solutions over your mobile device. The problem comes in the form of, even if they can, should they? What if they lose their device? What if it's infected with malware and now a Trojan is reporting information back? Because of this, you need to consider security for privacy, especially when a healthcare system is your primary client. Patient data and security is of the utmost concern and priority.

Controls and auditing are also important when dealing with the cloud provider. Managing a cloud system requires us to make sure that it's operating as it should. A correct management of a cloud system also means using elasticity correctly and decommissioning systems we no longer need or use. One of the biggest challenges with going to a cloud provider is that we get caught up in what we think are cost savings, but forget to practice correct processing, which leaves unused and forgotten systems online. You pay for that, so you need to have a process that audits and controls within your plan. Liaisons, such as the BRMs or service lines, can assist with that, or if your healthcare system has its own audit, risk, or compliance team, they can help as well.

MANAGING SYSTEMS FROM THE CLOUD WITH AIOps

We have spent some time focusing on how to deploy the systems and AIOps platform to the cloud. In the next section, I will show you how to manage your systems from the cloud. Conversely, I will also briefly explain how to use your internal AIOps system to manage your system in the cloud.

You need to consider a few caveats that can be easy to identify based on the network landscape, the size and complexity of your organization, its network and geographical layout, how the network connects everything, and what level of service you have with your cloud provider. Here are some considerations you should take a look at when trying to use AIOps in a cloud:

- Cloud adoption is generally based on a hybrid cloud environment.

- Managing the systems you host in a cloud environment with your AIOps solution depends on whether your cloud provider allows you to and on what it allows according to your contractual obligations.

There are many risks in this type of scenario, so you should consider its complexity and consider leveraging it if your cloud provider has its own way of providing event management and/or AI solutions.

Cloud Management and Monitoring Solutions

The basics have been covered, and now you are ready to manage your platform. Whether it's the base system of event and fault management or you have completed your deployment, gathered data over time, conducted analysis, and created intelligent workflows and automation (manually or dynamically), you are ready to do the same from the cloud. Cloud management/monitoring solutions are managed the same way you would any other system barring all of the caveats already mentioned.

Getting feeds/reports/dashboards like those shown in Figure 7.6 is no different than if you were monitoring the systems internally. Access to this dashboard may be different based on your design and deployment.

For example, you may need to log in via a console portal from the Web based on a universal URL (or web address) that your provider gives you.

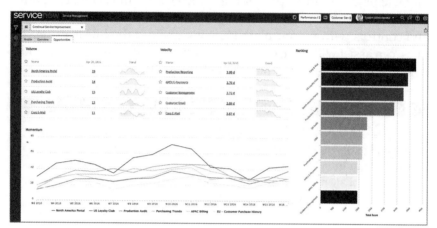

Figure 7.6: ServiceNow dashboards and reports in the Cloud

There may be some other ways to access the systems via a Citrix client or some other form of application provided by the cloud provider. The Dynatrace cloud can be accessed via a network portal. Figure 7.7 shows the accessibility of Dynatrace over the cloud from a portal.

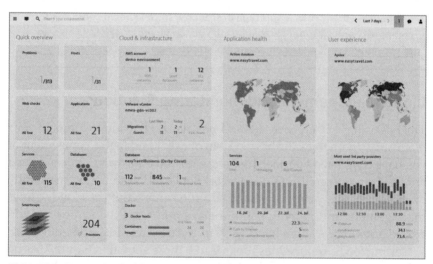

Figure 7.7: Dynatrace dashboard accessed via the cloud

Every cloud-based solution you deploy will be managed over a network of some kind. This requires you to be (or have the expertise of) a network architect and have someone (or a team) who can help you navigate other issues such as, what happens if you have Internet access problems? What if your name resolution for your company via the Domain Name System (DNS) service fails and you cannot resolve URLs or web addresses? What if the firewall rules get screwed up via a change and they block access to the portals you use? What if the systems cannot report in and you get thousands of false positive tickets supported to the help desk from access list problems? There are so many scenarios to consider, so having a great network as an asset is critical to your deployment success, especially over the cloud. A well-developed AIOps platform is designed to handle issues such as automating failover, alerting to issues, coming up with suggested responses, and so on, but you need people who understand these matters to ensure that your system is properly meeting your needs.

Summary

You are likely going to deploy AIOps into the cloud, use a cloud solution, or manage a cloud solution at some point, especially with the need for healthcare systems to spin up and spin out development systems, test systems, applications, and other technology that is not cost effective to do internally.

As you strategize and deploy AI operations into your healthcare setting, some of the most important considerations to take into account are where you will be hosting your platform and what type of service you will select if choosing the cloud. If you are choosing ServiceNow and ITOM, it's likely you will get to use their preset SaaS solution, or you may decide to deploy Splunk within an IaaS solution. Either way, this chapter armed you with the design information you need to have to intelligently set up AIOps and deploy it to serve those needs correctly and within budget.

This chapter helped you determine whether and how to move to the cloud by using real-world knowledge and experience. Whether you set your vendors on the request for proposal (RFP) process to get those answers, or, as a business relationship manager (BRM), you work with internal service lines to design the correct strategy—either way, you now have the ability to generate solutions that meet the needs of the business and the technology team as well as the clinicians who must use and rely on the technology you support. I discussed various challenges of cloud systems, including costs, preparation, deployment, migration, hybrid solutions, security, and privacy.

This chapter discussed how to consider the use of the cloud when deploying your AIOps system in a healthcare environment and, regardless of vendor choice, how you can be ready to deploy and manage, access, and control these assets correctly in an AIOps environment. Many professionals struggle with correctly planning this, especially when dealing with the complexity of a healthcare environment, and this chapter has shown you what is needed to do this successfully.

In the next chapter, we boldly explore the emerging world of AI, ML, and AIOps technologies in a healthcare environment.

The Future of Healthcare AI

"The future depends on what you do today."
—Mahatma Gandhi

As you strategize and deploy AI operations (AIOps) into your healthcare setting, all of the work you did in planning, strategizing, designing, and preparing should have provided you with a great product or solution that has helped you to gain valuable insight into the data you collect so you can trend, analyze, and look into predictive analytics. Workflow and automation should have provided you with a more efficient operational platform with some self-healing capabilities and event or fault handling that increased your ability to keep your technology up and running when the clinicians need it most. The future of healthcare AI, ML, and AIOps rests solely on what you do next in an ever-changing and evolving field of data capture, storage, analysis, and manipulation. Today you begin to look at the new technologies, workflows, techniques, solutions, services, and innovations that you can leverage based on big data and collected analytics. Today you can begin dreaming about tomorrow.

This chapter discusses the use of artificial intelligence (AI), machine learning (ML), and healthcare operations in an IT setting that leverages not only AIOps but other technologies and solutions as well. As we will see, much of how healthcare is delivered is constantly evolving and dynamically (and sometimes radically) in a state of flux and change. When the worldwide coronavirus (COVID-19) pandemic struck, it changed much of what we thought business as usual looked like. With mandatory quarantine, fear, and trying to control hospital surge, much of the healthcare and technology landscape changed overnight. In this chapter, I'll talk about that event, the technology in use, how the technology was changed, and the use of telemedicine, IoT, and other technologies that abruptly brought the future of AI, healthcare, and technology into the present. I will also talk about where AI was heading, how that has changed, and where we're heading now. The possibilities will be brought to light regarding what we as leaders, technologists, and healthcare professionals can do to realize this new world of technology that works for us, with us, and in some cases before us.

The Dynamically Changing World of AI

The future of AI in general and its fusion with machine learning, artificial intelligence, workflow automation, technology innovation, and big data all form a nucleus for everything we do in the world moving forward. We are emerging into a world of mobile handhelds where tons of data is consumed, created, stored, and saved for decades. What does that mean for the future? It means that all of that stored data can be used at some point and analyzed for whatever reasons that we may need or want. The sky becomes the limit on what we can achieve with big data. As long as the data is public and it's allowed to be accessed and used, we could learn an incredible amount from it.

In healthcare it's different. The data is mostly private and cannot be shared with others. Because of this restriction, it is hard to conduct research and do what could be effortless work with large amounts of incredibly helpful data unless you have explicit access and permission to use that data. In some cases, the data is stripped of personally identifiable information (PII) or protected health information (PHI). This is the information that connects the data to the actual person whom the data is representing. PHI is the cornerstone of how big data and healthcare analytics are handled in healthcare systems. Without it, we would not be able to use the EMR correctly; however, with it, we are cornered on our ability to use the data as a whole. With the removal of this information from the data, we can then use it in the same way we would use the aforementioned data that is public.

REFERENCE PHI is sometimes also referenced as personal health information. This data contains personally identifying information to the medical data such as name, location, home address, gender, and many more personal pieces of information or criteria. Other information includes (but is not limited to) demographics, test and lab results, conditions, and medical history, which if tied directly to the person would open up legal and ethical issues if used.

Think of your own private information. Would you want anyone looking through it for any reason at all besides those to whom you entrust your healthcare like your doctors and those who are sworn to protect it? We also need to consider the ethics and legality of using data in any aspect. Although way beyond the scope of this book and AIOps, it is worth mentioning that there are serious legal implications for the access and use of personal information without the knowledge or consent of those whom it represents.

So what does the future bring? As the old adage states, you need to know where you have been to know where you are going. If you do not know where technology has brought us until now, you will miss where we are going with it in the future. Much like the onset of virtual machines and cloud computing, AI-enabled systems are the technology that has been in development for years and that spawned from the need to be able to better utilize big data.

Figure 8.1 shows an undated timeline of where we started with the collection of massive amounts of data and what we intend to do with it and how the technology and the workforce needed to mature with it. Let's consider each point on that timeline.

- Large-scale growth, collection, and use of data were inevitable. As the commoditization of technology grew and the IoT expanded, we found ourselves with much more data and the ability to collect than ever before. In the early 1990s a SIMM memory chip cost a lot of money for a mere 8MB of RAM. Now, you can get terabytes of storage on a thumb drive you can order and receive from an online vendor in literally 24–48 hours. We originally took old pictures and scanned them or digitized old VHS tapes and made them into DVDs. Now we have mobile devices that can take and collect terabytes of data per person daily and upload to a cloud seamlessly. The exponential growth of data, and its collection and storage, is just unbelievable in 20+ years' time.

- New supporting technologies needed to be developed to allow for not only the collection but also the use of this large-scale growth of data. Big data was coined and so was the development, design, and deployment of storage area networks (SANs) that allowed for the access and use of a large-scale amount of data stored and sequenced in high-volume databases (DBs) and storage platforms.

- New AI and ML developments were created based on the growing size and use of data, but also its availabilities on the SAN and within the DBs. As the data grew and the ability to store and access it grew, so did the technology around it to manipulate and use the data. This is where analytics started to grow and become more and more valuable.

- The development of newer AI/ML tools began to spring up, and the prediction that just about every single piece of software, operating system, or service would be both cloud and AI enabled began to take hold. This is where the AIOps platforms began to spawn and become more and more approachable to the organizations that wanted to leverage this technology. Obviously, this is an AIOps-focused book in a healthcare environment; however, this is where any other tool, development system, platform, or function for AI and ML started to really take hold and become a bigger part of any technology or software release now and in the future.

- The next two items in Figure 8.1 bring us to the current day. The first is adding AI and ML skillsets to the modern workforce. This is where a book like this becomes extremely valuable. Now you can start to arm yourself with the knowledge of being able to deploy an AI/ML solution accurately and successfully.

- Finally, once you have a workforce enabled to do the work, you can test, pilot, strategize, deploy, and use an AI/ML (AIOps) solution in your organization, which is what the first seven chapters of this book focused on.

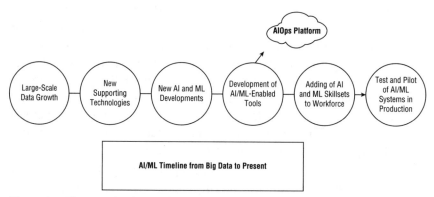

Figure 8.1: The growth of AI and ML

Current data shows us somewhere between the development of AI/ ML tools, building on older skillsets into new ones where AI and ML are a priority, and the development of these systems into our production environment. There is much to learn in this area, and this book looked to close the gap on that section of Figure 8.1's timeline when discussing how to deploy a tool (platform) like AIOps into your healthcare organization. Today's healthcare systems are growing rapidly, as is technology. For example, the IT team in healthcare today needs to keep pace with the technologies that are developing but also ensure that there is no disruption to current technologies that keep the clinical staff operational. To bridge that gap, there is a lot of planning and strategy that takes place. There are a lot of processes that need to be followed, and legal, HR, security, and many other groups such as application groups, clinical leadership, IT leadership, and others need to weigh in on how AI and ML work within their functions both separately and as a whole.

That is the basis of the future that you can plan. There may be unforeseen events and scenarios that you cannot plan for (for example, a specific pandemic, unanticipated legislation that changes the industry, or a sudden technological breakthrough that changes how your systems work), but most things can be strategized and developed over time. The future brings many new challenges to AI and ML, and as we saw with the coronavirus pandemic in 2020, everything can suddenly change in just a moment. This underscores that even the best strategy needs to have a contingency plan and be adaptable. You need to know what to do when things do not go as planned. Similarly, many of the technologies we use need to adapt to focus on telemedicine, remote access of systems, and usage of new applications that allow for different ways to access, use, find, and engage in clinical care, and there will definitely be new changes to AI and ML in developing these changes. Let's talk about what the future of AI brings regardless of a pandemic but also, because of it, ways we have had to make adjustments globally in every aspect of our lives, including how that directly affects not only AI and ML but also AIOps and the tools we look to deploy.

In 2020, the coronavirus (COVID-19) pandemic quickly spread across the globe and caused millions of cases of the disease to surface that overwhelmed many healthcare systems worldwide. Some of the protocols put in place by governments were to create restrictions by closing the economy, limiting movement of people, creating social distancing, and implementing cleanliness guidelines. These were just some of the many changes that rippled across governments, industries, and organizations. Some of the resulting changes to systems and AI relate more directly than others to the world of healthcare. This chapter will explore some of the more relevant developments.

The Future of AI

When we consider the future of AI, we also need to look at its past. Some history needs to be examined to learn lessons that can be applied to developing something for the future. We also need to look at trends, market disrupters, innovations, and so on. Some of the recent disrupters obviously were related to the coronavirus pandemic; however, there are many others. Had there not been a pandemic to deal with, there would still have been a different challenge to overcome. What made the pandemic unique is that it happened to affect the world of healthcare specifically and included many disrupters such as the following:

- **Budgets:** With the sudden arrival of the coronavirus, many organizations had to immediately consider how they were to make a living moving forward. Although you may think that healthcare is a bulletproof industry that cannot sustain financial devastation during a medical emergency, it's actually quite the opposite. Many of the areas where healthcare systems make money and build on their financial strengths (such as elective surgeries as an example) were put on hold so that surge units could be built and deployed.

- **Focus and priority:** The secondary disrupters were focus and priority, which put current projects on hold and focused all assets on developing ICU and ED space for the surge of patients. This required new construction and, in many cases, the use of new technologies.

- **New technologies and innovation:** The continued need to social distance brought a downward trend to the peak and downing curve of the coronavirus's surge. However, we needed to be vigilant for a potential re-surge. This required all of the surge developments to remain in place or be quickly mobilized as needed. It also created a demand for developing new technologies and procedures for a socially distanced medical experience. This brought in new ways to space (and limit) those who seek care and the explosion of telehealth and telemedicine and remote technology applications in the clinical space.

As shown in Figure 8.2, the grouping of all three challenges can be viewed as challenges that create positive outcomes. Current challenges to the healthcare systems and the development of AI and ML have all become opportunities. For example, today there is a focus on telemedicine and remote access.

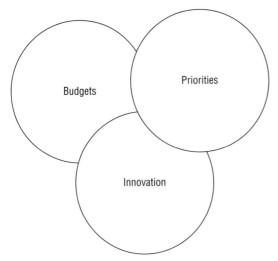

Figure 8.2: Current challenges to AI/ML

Because of this challenge, we are able to focus resources on the development and rapid build of remote-access technologies that were not a priority over other initiatives in the past. Some of these may not have received funding or were constantly reprioritized as low priority. Now, these new technologies can receive focus and, from there, give the clinicians more clinical abilities to reach patients and more freedom and flexibility for patients to receive healthcare. There is always a light at the end of the tunnel based on your perception of how to handle issues.

There are unavoidable and unfortunate setbacks based on priority, however. All of this causes strain on AIOps, but that does not mean that you cannot get things done, and it does not mean that you should put AIOps projects on hold. The AIOps platform is increasingly valuable for several reasons. For one thing, AIOps reduces the rates of existing outages, but it also provides the predictive usage of the system to prevent outages. It monitors the performance of the systems and allows self-healing to take place to ensure that the systems remain not only up and operational, but also at a capacity that allows clinicians to do their best work with a high level of availability.

Needed more now than ever are stable systems that are immediately fixed once they are seen as a fault or an event takes place. We can no longer see medical practices unable to access the EMR, telemedicine units unable to access their screens, or entire hospitals offline due to a series of system errors. The stakes are higher than ever now that we rely so much on healthcare more than ever before.

This is also the case for general AI and ML. Being used in industries other than healthcare, improved ML algorithms allow for analyzing of results through both supervised and unsupervised learning, and that output can be used to render better outcomes. The importance of this cannot be understated with current events in healthcare managing the health of millions around the globe. We need more deep learning of the data to help research teams find answers to questions that they otherwise cannot answer, particularly when it comes to understanding symptoms, risk factors, treatment contraindications, emerging techniques, and so on during a major pandemic. This need is transferable across any and every technology, industry, and service that exists today, and it is why AI and ML become hypercritical to everything we do now and in the future.

> **NOTE** Supervised learning is where you guide the machine how to perform its functions using clearly identified data. Unsupervised learning is where you let the machine learn from the data without requiring your direct guidance.

> **NOTE** The coronavirus pandemic was a major disrupter that sparked innovations, changes, and everything you can think about to reform the landscape of how business is done. Because of this, much of AI and ML experienced a change, but also a renewal of sorts. We can now look at research differently with a focus on leveraging AI and ML as a way to help move the process along faster and to get to positive results sooner. Consequently, AI/ML is used to scan millions of sections of data to help find potential treatments or cures (www.the-scientist.com/news-opinion/ai-is-screening-billions-of-molecules-for-coronavirus-treatments-67520).

Artificial Intelligence and Healthcare Innovation

AI and ML are not only innovations in themselves, but they mathematically help to create more innovations. AI and ML are an experiment in exponential growth of a technology unto itself. The more that is invested in ML, the more mathematically it can output. The more that is invested in the use of AI, the more innovation is derived based on the current product or service that is redeveloped using this technology.

The future of healthcare innovation and the use of AI and ML is focused on three major areas, and that is in the world of big data and analytics (or informatics), AIOps, and the use of telemedicine. In today's setting, large companies such as Microsoft, Google, Apple, Amazon, and just about every other major technology company are making, taking, and placing large-size bets on artificial intelligence and the use of machine learning fused into all of their offerings. Most of these offerings are also cloud hosted. Every one of these companies also specifically offers a healthcare offering, and some companies like Google are interested in becoming a healthcare company that can leverage AI and ML based on big data collected through their search engines as well as DNA collection. Google DNA collection and sequencing, identification, and use of big data are all next steps for the company to grow its footprint into the future. All the major players are on board and have their toes in the water while some have completely dived in. All other smaller fish have followed suit and are building out AI platforms and moving into the healthcare support space.

> **NOTE** Research and development (R&D) in these spaces is just as explosive in the healthcare organizations that handle clinical work. For example, most large healthcare systems have a research arm, usually affiliated with local colleges and other healthcare systems research teams.

Big Data, DataOps, Analytics, and Informatics

Big data collection and usage is one of the most significant innovations for our world. Although there are those who distrust or even fear it, the collection and usage of data to solve problems in medicine is critical to our survival. When we consider the future of AI and ML, we consider the processing of big data for the answers and trends we can see within it. This is where professional medical informatics specialists come in: they look through the data as it presents and determine what can be analytically derived from it. The more we join together and share information, the easier it will be to come to positive conclusions and outcomes. As we consider data transformation and usage and how that relates to outcomes, we need to also understand that AIOps covers the operations aspects of your data, but the true analytics are covered under the concept of DataOps, which is a data analytics philosophy poised to revolutionize data analytics in the same way DevOps revolutionized code development.

The AIOps platform is the central place that keeps the integrity of all applications, systems, services, infrastructure, and technology always on and available. This is where your lead systems engineers are looking for trends in the data to show concerns within operational aspects. When looking for trends in the data itself, DataOps is where you will find trend analysis information. This is also where automation and dynamic learning takes place to create a process workflow that makes sense and brings AI and self-healing alive. Once these steps have been taken, then the real magic begins. Make no mistake, AI is a large-scale transformation change to how organizations do business, and all large-scale companies and business are getting involved.

The clinical impact of AIOps can be seen in the forming of larger conglomerates to leverage technology and data to conduct intelligence operations and information analysis through ML to make automated decisions and ultimately identify trends in the data so it can be used in a positive way with automated workflows. An example we may all be aware of in today's modern healthcare systems is the use of an entire health system's data trending to identify population health challenges such as what diseases may be prevalent in certain areas. Without the collection and analysis of this data, we would not be able to make this prediction based on data and the trends it shows us. Although this book does not fully focus on these types of trends and their outcomes, AIOps allows for clinical operations performance improvements to become a reality.

The benefits of AIOps in the clinical space should not be underestimated. Without a fully running technology operation including the database systems that collect the data, stored on the large-scale storage systems that house the databases to the servers that deliver this information to the networks that connect it all together, there is no way that clinical operations and AI can exist without the use of AIOps solutions in your technology operations space. AIOps make sure that the systems remain in a high state of uptime and availability through event monitoring and automated workflow for self-healing. The increase of data storage and analytics places strains on system performance, and AIOps can help achieve increased efficiencies and system uptime. That said, let's look at how each of these cross over to make both solutions a reality in your organization and why both serve each other and create a symbiotic relationship.

Another interesting concept of big data, information collection, analytics, informatics, AI/ML, and AIOps is the focus on crowdsourcing. Crowdsourcing is simply providing the data of many for the usage by one. So for example, if you make data accessible by many to use and analyze, you have created a crowdsource on big data. See Figure 8.3. In an MIT article (news.mit.edu/2017/crowdsourcing-big-data-analysis-1030) where crowdsourcing was used to leverage big data to create better technology, the outcomes were significant. FeatureHub, which was inspired by GitHub, is an online repository of open-source programming projects and massively popular among developers who create innovative ideas daily. It had thousands of contributors partake in a competition to get more contributors on the system. The outcome (like many crowdsourcing

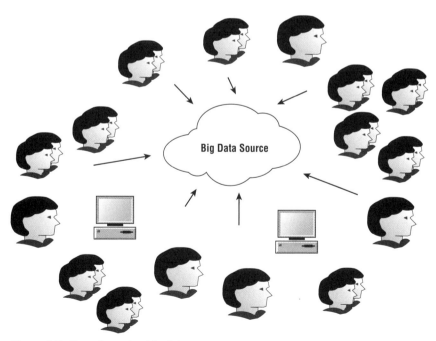

Figure 8.3: Crowdsourcing big data

solutions) was that you had a greater number of smart people crunching information that was collected (big data) to get to a conclusion. Obviously, when more people and devices feed information into big data, that provides more data for AI and ML to work with, proportionally improving all AI-related efforts. This further helps researchers, clinicians, and other users more effectively use both the AI and the big data in a myriad of ways.

The crowdsource can be a control group or a public group that may be uncontrolled. This plays into the science of the predicted and solution-based outcomes; however, that goes beyond the scope of this book. What we want to focus on is that the use of big data is here to stay. The use of this data is what propels us into the future, and whether it be a tool or a group of users crunching the data, you work to get to an outcome that presents trends, findings, or outcomes from the data you are working with. I think that finding cures to a virus that causes a pandemic is likely one of the best examples of using big data today.

NOTE   The future of crowdsourcing is bright. Once more security can be applied and controls are in place, not only we can crowdsource with people, but we can also crowdsource with tools, which directly feeds into how people and AI working together can further leverage big data for their needs. This does create its own challenges, but imagine a world where data is safely shared to solve problems across the world. I can imagine it and predict that one day we will be there.

Telehealth (Telemedicine)

Telemedicine is the delivery of healthcare services to patients through the use of "tele" technology. The word is derived from telephone or telecommunications, but it's simpler than that. Think network connection or Internet. Telemedicine allows for services to be delivered via electronic communication technologies for the ability to connect patients to experts to provide clinical support.

Since the arrival of the coronavirus, nothing has been more important than telemedicine in the work of healthcare. Because of this, the future of AI, ML, and AIOps must firmly sit with the ability to provide medical, clinical, and technical support from anywhere in the world. As predictive analytics from big data help to guide patient care in a way that allowed clinicians and providers to offer solutions (and additional services as well) to those in need, it is based on results gleaned from past similar treatments. That same mentality is fused now with telemedicine where the ingested data is also incorporated in the form of who is now using telemedicine and why. Doctors and clinicians work with tests, patient histories, and lab results at the click of a button. It is becoming increasingly common for patients to access their doctors and lab results through a portal or over their phone or other devices, reducing the number of in-person consultations. Figure 8.4 shows the ease of use, simplicity, and flexibility that telehealth brings to the consumer by consulting with their physician from even a mobile device.

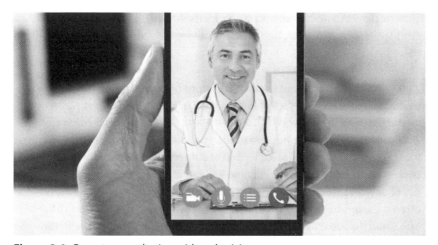

Figure 8.4: Remote consultation with a physician

Although modern telehealth and telemedicine has been around for more than two decades, the coronavirus pandemic pushed them into the forefront of healthcare services, and they are now a need instead of a want. The disrupters to create future innovation in AI were brought to our doorstep in 2020 courtesy of the coronavirus pandemic.

There was a demand to be able to provide telemedicine to patients immediately. With millions of people around the country encouraged to stay home and worried about potentially exposing themselves to the virus, many of them turned to telemedicine companies. According to the US Centers for Disease Control and Prevention, telemedicine became an even more essential service required to keep people healthy. Telemedicine companies stepped in to give patients a chance to talk through their symptoms and determine whether they need to be hospitalized.

The need for social distancing drove a much wider adoption of contactless testing, remote consultations, and using portals to transmit data, and this is only likely to continue to grow in the future. When these technologies are unified in an AIOps system, the data provided through them can immediately feed into the AI and ML functionality, strengthening and speeding up the entire process.

This becomes a game changer, and the ability to keep this service up and running is where AIOps will become a critical player in event, fault-and self-healing technologies required to keep these systems up and running. The future of healthcare AI is now, and the requirements have been expanded. Putting telemedicine into safe, secure, well-kept, integrity-based infrastructures that do not suffer performance degradation or downtime has become a priority for AIOps. The next phase of digital transformation for health systems starts with remote capabilities for all clinical support.

NOTE   People sometimes draw distinctions between telemedicine, telehealth, and telecare. The care provided from a clinician to a patient via an interaction over the network and using these tools is called *telemedicine*. *Telehealth* is the overarching term used to provide similar services but in a passive capacity through the collection of data from biomedical (biomed) devices that supply active information without intervention or through the use of devices that are self-managed or monitored. Another term used less often is *telecare*, which is the management of health and the providing of care using the proactive methods of managing the delivery of care with the use of technology. Obviously, there is some overlap between these terms, and it is common for people to use them interchangeably.

Telehealth Innovations

As we continue to expand on the current model of telehealth and incorporate it into the fabric of everything we do, we need to apply a continued focus on how to support it. Some of the predicted technologies that we will need to develop and support in healthcare environments are the applications and application health of bots, security, high-level video usage, more provider support, and expanded options to monitor and manage the environment.

When we consider how we will expand the use and management of telemedicine, we need a way to get the right people to the right care without a large amount of red tape. AI will help with that triage and request (like an old phone call tree) of integrated logic that allows the routing and connecting of calls to the correct places of care in the clinical setting. AI if used correctly can track previous requests and allow for future requests to follow the same patterns and thus paths that were used before. This speeds up care. Another helpful innovation is to focus on how to use video in a way that it does not impact our network, Internet, infrastructure, and other systems or create a performance hit. High levels of video traffic without the correct use of compression and routing or prioritization with queuing can cause massive problems on current infrastructures. Think about the old IP phone deployments that required a lot of focus to get calls to be 100% reliable when we departed the traditional telecommunication analog-based technologies for today's digital ventures. This is something that we need to predict, counter, and be ready for with the growing number of users in this space. AIOps can be used to leverage this infrastructure and start to self-heal by applying dynamic failover to less used systems, alternate paths that are less congested, and other methods to provide more acceptable performance.

Another avenue where healthcare, telehealth, biomed, and AIOps can all converge is on the self-managed biomedical devices that are either on-premise or at home. As more remote home service begins to take hold, telemedicine and telehealth services need to expand but also be manageable and monitored for health. The health of the system is just as critical as the health of the patient it is trying to care for. It's an interconnected system where there is a need for all of the components to be connected and usable. AIOps can help in this area by providing fault management notification through incident triage of any outage or performance challenge the system may take.

As a use case, consider the home of a diabetic patient who is ill and must be monitored for health. They need to submit information via their pump or sensors into the system so that a telemedicine visit can be configured and set up to discuss patient numbers. Telehealth via the biomedical devices that are connected to the system over the network to the core network of the healthcare system must remain operational and safe. Any fault to the system must be reported in real time and have an incident or problem acknowledged and handled immediately. This is a realistic situation that, although it is a simple use case, probably maps to hundreds if not thousands of people who may have their health managed this way in the coming years. Any mistakes in this chain could cause corruption of data and incorrect care procedures. In some cases, with other diagnoses, the timeliness of support could mean life or death.

If we want to consider what the infrastructure would look like in a telehealth (telemedicine) AIOps blueprint, we can visualize this in Figure 8.5. Here we can envision that we have a healthcare system that has a datacenter with infrastructure managed and monitored via a cloud-based AIOps platform for event and fault management. There are biomedical devices and systems connected to the corporate network, and all systems are managed via the AIOps platform. The healthcare system offers telehealth and telemedicine options via the patient portal that is accessible over the Internet either via desktop, private kiosk, or mobile device. Here, the appointment can be made, and all of the interconnection can be managed and maintained via the portal. Most importantly, the health of the entire system is handled by AIOps. The example I want to use here is if there was a problem with a corrupted index on the database of a system that caused issues with the entire telehealth platform. Because the system is managed via the AIOps platform, it was identified and corrected in real time using automation and alerting of issues in real time. Because of this, the patient's vitals were not corrupted, and the clinicians were able to provide care without any interruption, disruption, or corruption of resources.

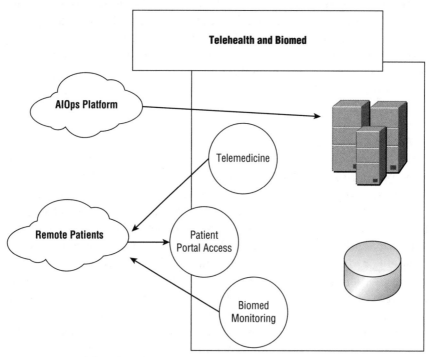

Figure 8.5: A telehealth and AIOps blueprint

CAUTION   Although an external cloud-based AIOps solution can work, you could implement an in-house one as well. This does bring to light possible concerns about moving to a cloud solution in a real use case scenario. If you chose to use the externally based cloud solution and did not size your Internet connection or all of your network and firewall devices correctly, the load of the now in-demand and immediately required telemedicine solutions with intensive video could tip your network links over the edge. Make sure you consider all of these scenarios before making your choice.

Telehealth AI

Now that we have examined the fundamentals of why remote access, remote services, telehealth, and telemedicine are the big disrupters and so important in healthcare systems today, we need to explore how all of this ties directly into AI and ML and why we need AI and ML as well as AIOps to be a big part of managing the overall technology as it evolves. AIOps is used to make sure that the overall usage of these technologies remains stable and available.

Telehealth AI is the incorporation of patient-generated data that has been cleared for use so that it can be collected, analyzed, and trended to find better ways to provide care. The review of health data in a way that allows for the streamlining of telemedicine consults, automation of routing of problems to different providers, automation and routing of lab and other pharmacy information, and innovation pre-screening and predictive determination of health diagnosis is where we want to take telehealth AI in the future.

In the future of telehealth, telemedicine and the incorporation of AI technology can be used for the intake and triage of patients. For example, consider the example of a lab engineer connecting remotely with a patient. This might look innocently like a standard video communication, as shown in Figure 8.6, but behind the scenes there are many possible areas of AI/ML integration that can come into play.

- Priority routing through a routing bot finds that the patient is in need of a consult immediately, and it does this through AI/ML to determine through the queue who may require special needs, attention, or prioritization.

- The initial connection with the patient finds that the patient speaks in a language that is not English. Because of this, an automated bot starts up to begin a translation.

- Throughout the dialogue there are markers that will create a pop-up alert if medical terminology is used and not understood. This can be further re-created into a knowledge base (KB) article that may be loaded in ServiceNow that can be pulled up and offered to the patient in the language of their choice based on current dialog taking place.

- As the consult is taking place, a bot is automatically launched that is silently doing the medical billing portion and filling out all of the medical billing codes for ICD-10 and other coding required for revenue cycle.

- A privacy scan bot has alerted that the end user is not in a silent, secure, or private location and generates an alert for both the provider and the patient that the patient information could be disclosed due to the lack of privacy.

- During the consult, the network connection was disrupted, and the AIOps platform performed a warm transfer of the connection to another server and network connection that allowed the state to be maintained and the connection to be reestablished within seconds.

- The notes in the EMR were autopopulated, and based on the keywords used, an after-care checklist was automatically pulled and sent via PDF to the patient portal for the patient's review.

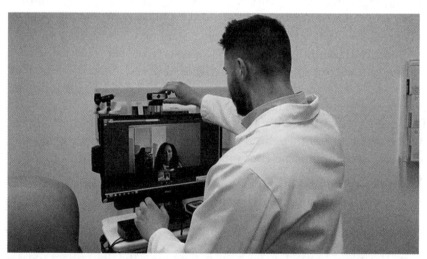

Figure 8.6: Using telehealth AI

I can go on and on and on. It's really "sky is the limit" with how we can develop and move into a new way of AI/ML supporting telehealth and telemedicine. As we move into the area of biomedical devices and how they interact as well as the IoT, we can expand AI even more deeply into what is possible. When we incorporate big data, the opportunities expand even more. Once we realize that bots and the use of machine learning can scan and filter through large quantities of data rapidly and accurately, we can create the ability to identify medical issues, diagnose, and even proactively treat issues before they occur. An example would be if someone's labs showed a pattern of cholesterol levels that were increasingly getting worse, it would make sure that the patient knew and was given advice on how to change those numbers, prescribe medication if needed, and continue to track and monitor the numbers based on the next blood labs that were done. If labs were not done in a specific timely threshold, an alert would be generated, and the patient and the clinician would be given the chance to be reminded that this was something that needed to be dealt with. In today's non-AI world, all of this relies on both the patient and the clinician reminding or recommending that these forms of action be taken. Because of this, it would be safe to say that AI is allowing us to make better decisions and, thus, better diagnoses. It allows us to reduce wait times and locations, removes transporting those who should not be moved, allows for access to highly trained and specialized experts as needed in your home, and allows for proactive solutions to give you better chances at good health.

With AI (and AIOps), the ability to do remote patient monitoring is crucial, especially during pandemics and other instances of limited physical access. When we are not able to access sick patients' rooms safely, AIOps allows us to be able to connect with them via remote devices and screens and provide care safely.

NOTE It should be noted that there is a big difference between providing care in person and doing telemedicine. Bedside manner, the human connection, and the building of trust are things that telemedicine struggles with. Although this is not a chapter on clinicians and how they interoperate with technology to provide their services, it is about providing care nonetheless, so if you are a clinician reading this, remember that people rely on the human connection, and it's hard to do that at times via a computer screen. Because of this, it's important to make sure that we consider emotions, psychology, and how we interact with our patients.

Future Innovation Merging Clinical and IT Operations

What is the future of AIOps and healthcare? Expansion and integration at an amazing pace. We will see the adoption of more and more AI/ML options in everything we use and do. That said, the importance of providing these services in the future with technology packages that allow for this innovation must be considered.

So, what do healthcare leaders want? Having been around many executive-level leaders in both IT and clinical operations, reducing costs is at the top of the list. We spend too much for less than what we predict. Also at the top of the list is making technology work for us, not against us. Allowing the clinical staff to focus on doing clinical work and not have to do notes, back-office work, documentation, and other administrative duties reduces the load on clinicians and gives them more opportunity to do clinical work and thus see more patients and focus on what they are experts in. Speaking to one doctor, the expansion of telemedicine is great because they can see more patients; however, the additional overhead is still there to make sure that all back-office procedures are completed. AI and ML seek to solve this. If the systems could be more intelligent based on collected data and experiences, they could help to offload this work and make technology more valuable.

Streamlining business operations equals streamlined healthcare services, and using technology to achieve this would be the overall goal. This is similar to clinical staff doing back-office work, but it can also map to other areas of the healthcare system that can be automated such as automated call routing and placement in queues. If a specialized treatment or consult is required, it can be mapped accordingly via technology, much like a supply chain. This can be further developed with ML and blockchain so that if a decision is made, we can reverse engineer it to understand why it was made and learn from the machine that is making the decisions.

TIP   The concept of blockchain comes up when we talk about business process rewriting and how to make AI work to better derive a streamlined workflow. The convergence of blockchain and AI help with this function.

Blockchain is the digital supply chain of the future. It is defined as a decentralized network of computers that records and stores data to display a chronological series of events on a transparent and immutable ledger system. It works hand in hand with AI and ML to store what is important and what to do with that information based on its value. When machine learning is in use, blockchain can store the data used and help to decode why a decision was made.

So, what does a helpful innovative chain of technology look like where the technology is doing all of the work behind the scenes? Figure 8.7 shows every technology we have spoken about in action where the center of all of the clinician support is AI and the overall blanket monitoring every single piece of technology in this diagram is AIOps.

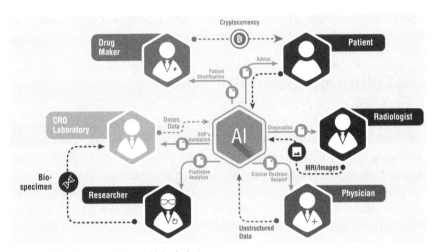

Figure 8.7: Using AI, ML, and blockchain

There are quite a few technology advancements working in this workflow that provide both business process and healthcare delivery services and processes to be fully automated and give the clinician the ability to do clinical work, making the expert focus on using the technology to their advantage instead of having it work against them creating more work for them to do.

- The physician (or any clinical provider) giving the consult via telemedicine is able to use AI throughout the entire process to do any other service required to include labs, radiology, payment, pharmacy, or other.

- The entire system is protected and monitored via the AIOps platform for performance and uptime, integrity, and availability. If any problem is detected anywhere in the system, it can be used as an event management tool to send a fault or event to create a ticket within the help desk automatically, which can be routed to a service technician or to an on-call technician on standby who can immediately take it. This is in addition to any self-healing or correcting capabilities.

- If any ML or AI function is not understood, it can be reviewed for process and workflow to ensure correctness.

This is a simple outlook on the possibilities. As we talk about what the future brings, there is much hope invested in the use of AI, ML, and blockchain. They could be developed into a more complete solution to deliver a synergistic impact when combined; however, today they are still being developed so that they can be used together more efficiently.

The Future and Beyond

The majority of what I have discussed up until now has been things that actually lurk on the horizon. Many of the things I mentioned have been conceptualized, planned, or even in development as possibilities for the future. There is much more we can learn about AI and ML and the possibilities they bring. However, there has also been decades of work on the topic and many interesting developments that have been released or implemented over the years.

The first topic of importance to consider is the actual product line expansion, integration, and innovations that we have discussed thus far in this book. This book has discussed ServiceNow, Splunk, and various other products and technologies that currently have the lion's share of the market, are Gartner Magic Quadrant winners, and in all honesty provide some of the best solutions on the market today. That said, these products and many of the other products all have the same thing in common. You. Your business is what they want, and you need to be wary of what you are sold. I cannot send you out hoping that there is a bright future when we are still living in the present and that present is showing us that AI in all of its glory is still hard to implement, costly, and risky in most instances.

If you really commit to performing this book's lessons well in laying out a good project plan, performing due diligence, selecting a system, and delivering services, you will do well. You will have a system that will provide you with great AIOps and many other needed benefits. Most if not all monitoring solutions are put in place to provide event and fault management. If your system goes down, it is unavailable, the disk drive fills up, the memory dumps, or the network link disconnects, you are going to know immediately. In most cases, the system will heal itself based on what the outage was. It could be someone made a mistake and corrected it on their own. It could be a provider lost service and impacted your system. There are many reasons why this can happen, and this base system is going to provide you with that level of protection needed and justified in any healthcare system (or any other type of business) today. The truth is, after that, everything else is additional programming. So, where does that leave us for the future?

For one, do not lose hope. I hope I shared enough in this book with you to show you how far we have come in a short period of time. With AI and ML advancements and how they integrate with every part of healthcare technology, AIOps is maturing at an ever-increasing rate. With new vectors such as telemedicine, there is room for growth. The ability to self-heal, which will reduce the overhead, reduce the footprint, and allow you to reduce costs, takes time to work out and is usually not a plug-and-play opportunity. It can't be, and you certainly do not want it to be in all instances. You do not want the system to think that a false positive is actionable and therefore shut down your entire datacenter for a period of time. That might be an alarming example, but I want you to really digest why it's important to understand that implementing AIOps will never fully be plug and play. Future deployments of these systems will have wizards and process templates that will allow you to more easily implement these services, but you should still plan on reviewing everything for accuracy regardless.

Newer versions of AIOps platforms will also become more feature rich with the ability to out-of-the-box implement and manage newer technologies like telemedicine, software-defined wide area network (or SD-WAN), cloud monitoring and management technologies, and more. They will also be able to work with bigger data, the bigger brother of big data. We all know data will continue to grow at a staggering rate, and the need to be able to manage it will continue to grow. Larger databases, more involved storage area networks (SANs), and the fabric that connects them will become more complicated, and the need to manage them will also be critical to keeping everything up and running.

In Figure 8.8, a home user uses a software-defined wide area network (SD-WAN) device to connect over the Internet securely and safely to a resource or to create a telemedicine session.

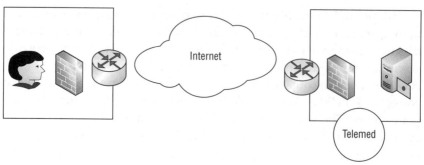

Figure 8.8: Understanding SD-WAN.

Open-source technologies may also begin to rise again. Back in the day closed source became disrupted by open source, and now you have both keeping pace. Most healthcare systems use closed-source technologies because the need to secure them is so great. However, the belief that closed source provides safer and more supportable products is under debate.

AI's other use cases also continue to grow. The advancement of converged systems needs to be considered as more and more mergers and acquisitions (M&A) activity takes place. In these instances, the costs to convert are extremely high and/or the operation cannot withstand an outage long enough to cost the provider large sums of income. Consequently, we see many dissimilar systems needing to connect and interact with each other. Advancement in converging systems and their proper management with AIOps will be more and more important as these systems develop.

We are already in the process of transitioning from the present into the future as the infrastructure of healthcare converges with the clinical aspect of providing care and using biomedical (biomed) devices. As we continue to change, adapt, and overcome challenges, the ability to manage and monitor these systems reliably and get them on a managed solution like AIOps becomes critical to providing needed care. This is especially true in the telehealth, biomedicine, and AIOps arenas. The patient experience is reimagined, and the consumer is the center of the universe in the new AIOps-driven world. As we move into home-based networks, remote office, and the need to provide anytime/anywhere access to users looking to gain service, we need to consider that AIOps needs to help deliver on that vision.

Robotic inclusion is another consideration for the future. The meeting of hardware and software with machine learning, AI, and all manageable data under the AIOps umbrella is a promising development. It could help bring asset management, inventory, and every component contained on the network into the event management arena. Robots and the AI/ML technology they use can also be considered for AIOps. Considering that both robotic process automation (RPA) and software-based robotics provide automation, could they be connected and used together? This could be one avenue of digital transformation that could be fused to add a new dimension to the ability to self-heal.

RPA can integrate and interact with AIOps tools to provide an additional scope to handling business and technology processes. There may be needs for robotic inclusion to do the following:

- Swap out failed hardware such as hard drives, RAID drives, tapes, or other FRUs
- Change tapes if still applicable
- Push buttons
- Connect cables
- Perform any other needed hands-on solution

If we used these two technologies together, we could imagine a world where you had an event correlation based on a failure of a device. For example, you got an alert that multiple drives failed an array and needed to be replaced. A ticket can be cut, and from there, the drives are gathered and replaced, and then the ticket is closed. While historically RPA has focused outside the IT landscape, we can see that there is a possibility for its use in the future.

The key to AIOps is that it is based on your infrastructure and its health. It's mostly internal, whereas RPA is more external. RPA has also been historically used to provide simple actions that are predefined and not based on dynamic workflow calculated from ML. RPA can also be software based and internal; however, they are still considered simple programs that follow a specific set of instructions. In the future, automation should meet with self-healing where AIOps, ML, and RPA can all provide a solution that allows the inclusion of hardware-based robotics to interact with software-based management systems to perform tasks outside the scope of the connected network and the technology that supports it.

It is unclear what the future of robotics, hardware, and other solutions merged or fused with AIOps will look like. However, the ideas are out there, and I hope to see some movement in the future in these areas to build on the AIOps platforms' abilities.

AIOps, the Cloud, and Security

The future of the cloud and the security required to handle AIOps appropriately in a healthcare system is another important topic to consider. Tomorrow's cloud is nothing more than a hybrid fusion of an organization's datacenter, a cloud provider (or multiple providers), remote home offices, remote offices, patients connecting to services, and the reliability of every one of the services offered by the organization.

The connectivity between all of these systems will be generally over secure connections via the Internet, and the service provided will be an offering of what you can get from the cloud and what you offer via your own datacenter. Security will be the most important concept for you to consider as a risk and liability. At any point in this chain an exposure can take place if any mistakes are made. Systems that grow too big too quickly become difficult to manage.

Tomorrow's AIOps needs to be an interconnected system that allows for flexibility but also for security and risk assessment. By allowing risk assessments to take place (like penetration tests) and security vulnerability scanning, you can assess threats and remediate them as you deploy.

Summary

This is the end of our journey together, but it marks the beginning of your journey as a knowledgeable and confident leader who can use AI, ML, and AIOps. Over the course of the book, you explored strategy and preparing, planning, and implementation, as well as the use and refinement of your enterprise solution. You examined many different platforms, including the most commonly used ones in the market today. You learned a lot about what makes the underlying infrastructure come to life and how to integrate your clinical systems and operations into a platform that allows you to automate and ideally work to eliminate downtime and outages in your priority environment. Working in healthcare can be a life or death situation, so keeping the EMR and other key systems such as the pharmacy, labs, the OR, the ED, and the ICU up and running at all times is critical.

As you strategize and deploy AIOps into your healthcare setting, all of the work you did in planning, strategizing, designing, and preparing should have provided you with a great product or solution that has helped you to gain valuable insight into the data you collect so you can trend, analyze, and look into predictive analytics. The big data collection should allow you to start to automate more intelligently and create outcomes that make sense. Workflow and automation should provide you with a more efficient operational platform with some self-healing capabilities and event or fault handling that increase your ability to keep your technology up and running when the clinicians need it most.

The future of healthcare AI, ML, and AIOps rests solely on what you do next in an ever-changing and evolving field of data capture, storage, analysis, and manipulation. Things are constantly changing for the healthcare field, as we saw with the coronavirus, which changed everything. This chapter explored the use of artificial intelligence (AI), machine learning (ML), and healthcare operations in an IT setting leveraging big data, innovative technologies such as telemedicine, and how AIOps can be used to interconnect all of it. The future truly does rest on how you take your solid foundation and continue to build on it. Today you begin to look at the new technologies, workflows, techniques, solutions, services, and innovations that you can leverage based on big data and collected analytics. Today you begin dreaming about tomorrow. Today you implement the future.

CHAPTER 9

The Convergence of Healthcare AI Technology

"To create greater convergence, we need more integration."
—**Emmanuel Macron**

The next phase of innovation comes from the convergence of technologies. As more technology is used to bolster processes, functions, and tasks we do every day, we run the risk of making things more complex than they need to be. Because of the fast rate of technological adaption and reliance on technology, it is critical to take a good hard look at what we can do as clinicians, leaders, healthcare innovators, and technologists to ensure that the future of medicine is delivered with more simplicity. The large-scale applications, programs, and systems that are deployed and managed are now being integrated at a fast-growing rate. All of this integration creates the convergence of systems and opportunities to scale the systems up but also out to create resiliency, more computing power, and essentially more flexibility to leverage systems as a whole for more insights. It is critical as AI progresses into the future and there is a need to manage it as a whole that we make sure that the AIOps platform is positioned to do just that.

This chapter discusses the use of artificial intelligence (AI), machine learning (ML), and healthcare operations in an IT setting that holistically leverages not only AIOps, but also other technologies and solutions. We want to consider the umbrella effect when we use AIOps. The more we are able to cover with AIOps, the better we will be at maximizing the full benefit of the growth of all integrated and converged systems as a whole. AIOps platforms can help you manage all of your disparate technologies from one central location. It also helps you take advantage of the Internet of Things (IoT), which is one of the largest growing technologies in healthcare information technology (HIT). IoT, AI, ML, and AIOps are playing a central role in the future success of delivering better healthcare by bringing together the integration and convergence of these technologies. For the beginning, we must learn what each of these disparate technologies is and how they can converge under one platform of managed services.

Overview of Convergence

We are starting this section by discussing the future of AI in general and how the fusion of machine learning, artificial intelligence, workflow automation, technology innovation, and big data all form a nucleus for everything we do in the world moving forward. In the previous chapter, we touched on what the future would bring to AIOps, and now we take that one step further to look at the future of how AI can converge with AIOps to create better clinical outcomes in healthcare systems that use this technology.

The most important part of the convergence equation is to understand who we are serving. There is nothing more important than the patient in clinical care. The entire healthcare system revolves around clinicians providing service to patients and their families. Everything that healthcare systems do (including the technology they use) is provided as a service to ensure that the primary mission of providing quality care is met and surpassed. Technology is at the forefront of this simple equation and ensures the infrastructure needed to create opportunities for delivering care in a connected world. We rely on technology for everything we do, so healthcare acting as a microcosm of our world is no different. In fact, the technology provided needs to not only be the best we can offer but also be dynamic enough to change rapidly with the needs of the clinician's work on a daily basis. As health innovation takes place, technology must be in line with (and sometimes ahead of) it to be useful. You could say that one cannot operate without the other these days, and therefore the need for convergence is critical to success. Integration of systems allows all parties to share technology to increase best-case outcomes for everyone involved.

Convergence brings technology and the needs of the clinician together to be used in a way where one technology helps to build upon the other. Once integration and convergence occur, AI can be used to help create opportunities where none existed before. Think of integration as the connection between disparate systems, and think of convergence as the synergy that takes place when these systems can be used together via configuration or shared services.

As these systems connect, they provide more value. We will even learn that what we try to do technically in the healthcare settings is an advanced version of what each of us may be trying to do in our own homes with smart home technology. Even more interesting is that our homes may become the new patient rooms extending the healthcare system even further over the Internet to connect everyone anywhere to access quality health services. This can give clinical staff the immediate response to those in need even if they haven't left their homes when in need. The following are some of the key areas to consider:

- **Patient monitoring and alerts:** This can be done with IoT, and it provides real-time alerting to monitoring staff who can react promptly. This can be done in a hospital or practice setting as well as in a home-based setting.

- **Equipment management, configuration, testing, calibration, and updating:** The constant monitoring of connected devices allows a centralized system that is AI-aware to automatically handle all of the needs of the IoT.

- **Data analysis and analytics:** This can be done on all devices connected to the centralized system to identify trends, abnormalities, or other positive (or negative) data that requires action. Action can be taken automatically based on ML.

NOTE The use of home-based technology and wearables driven by the IoT gives access to immediate alerting, which can be critical in saving time in responding to life-threatening circumstances. IoT devices can gather data and transfer it to doctors in real time. They can track what is required to provide care as well as give and send alerts to those who need to know. The use of AI can help to automate, filter, and process this data as well as prioritize or send it to specific groups as required.

Note that Figure 9.1 shows a very high-level overview of what an integrated (and converged) healthcare system (services, technology, IoT devices and functions) looks like when AI and HIT are connected, shared, and leveraged together as one. Here, the AIOps platform can manage all devices that are connected no matter what they are or where they are. If they are connected and configured in the AIOps platform, they can be managed, mapped, alerted on, data collected, backed up, and even automated to self-heal if needed.

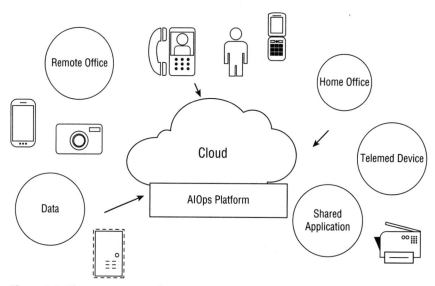

Figure 9.1: The convergence of AI and HIT

To get to this point, systems need to be integrated. There are many ways you can plan this and add it to your project plan for AIOps deployment.

- When deploying AIOps, you need to know what systems will be added to the event and fault management, alerting, and incident triage process. By adding these systems, you have created an integration point. A good example would be when you want your network infrastructure to be connected to the AIOps platform. For fault management, you can set the Simple Network Management Protocol (SNMP) strings in the devices so that the AIOps platform, routers, or switches can connect, integrate, and work together. Once completed, if the switch experiences an issue (for example, it overheats), it can send an alert to the AIOps platform so that it can be triaged and handled. Once the two systems are connected and work in a way where a ticket is cut and handled, or self-healing is done via dynamic automation, you have a converged system.

- Consider an example where you have all of your remote telemedicine carts managed via the AIOps platform remotely. If any problem takes place in any of the carts (for example, a dead or failing battery), it can send an alert to the AIOps system. Having the carts' system integrated with the AIOps system allows the systems to proactively alert each other. If properly leveraged, they can also self-heal (perhaps switch to a different battery or cart).

The convergence of systems can bring about many benefits and increased value. However, without the systems interconnected and working together, you cannot leverage the benefits of convergence. For example, if a temperate threshold for a device reached a critical point, if nothing was done, it would ruin the component or device and render the system inoperable. In some cases, you may have to replace a component to get the system back up and running. Now, let's consider that this system was a critical piece of equipment used to provide care. More importantly, what if the device was so critical that it was used to power other systems in an operation room (OR), and if the system was lost, it could cause the inability to operate? This is why healthcare information technology (HIT) and the use of AIOps can provide critical services to keep other lifesaving services up and running.

WARNING   "Convergence of systems" is a hot topic and one that needs to be considered to better increase benefits and reduce complexity. However, there is one place where complexity could be increased, but it needs to be considered prior to the deployment of any integrated and shared systems. Security of converged systems can become more complex based on what is being integrated. For example, make sure that patient information is shared only with those who are meant to see it. An example would be if you started to join systems and some of them had access to PHI or PII. If that is the case, you should involve security experts to make sure that there are no exposure points of any kind.

Systems Integration

The integration of systems can be complex. When we consider infrastructure, most systems are made to integrate without too much effort. Planning takes the most time to ensure that everything is done correctly, but most systems are made to join with other systems fairly easily. This is also even more prevalent when you are working with limited vendors. For example, if you are working primarily with Microsoft and use Microsoft technologies, it's a good bet that all of it will integrate (and converge) quite easily. The best example of this is with Microsoft Office products and Office 365. With Microsoft Teams and other available products, you can now cloud-host all of your applications, which can be used together without much effort. When considering an infrastructure like domain name resolution with the Domain Name System (DNS) and directory services (Active Directory), it's likely that once you roll the systems out, they will easily integrate. The challenge comes when you start to look at dissimilar systems and how they may be connected. Another example would be with services and applications. Many times, applications need to be configured to work with other applications and require additional programming (or coding) to accomplish this task. You need to keep in mind all of these aspects when you plan the connection and use of all shared systems and services.

The configuration and interconnection of network and server systems create the backbone services of your entire technical architecture. This enables your service and applications to run on top of them and be grown as platforms. These services and applications can also be interconnected. For example, your basic electronic medical record (EMR) software can be used by clinicians to access a patient's records from any kiosk, host, desktop, laptop, smartphone, or mobile device that was authorized to provide such access. Now, there will be other systems that tie into that EMR such as blood lab systems, radiology and imaging systems, and pharmacy applications. All of these also integrate into systems that handle the revenue cycle and other billing and patient scheduling software systems.

REFERENCE   Sometimes it is hard to imagine how many interconnected systems there are in a healthcare system as it truly is a massive undertaking to provide a full spectrum of services via technology. Picture archiving and communication system (PACS) is the basic building block of today's medical imaging technology used to share, review, and analyze radiology images. The requirements for such a system are usually massive in that some of these high-slice image files can be extremely large to save, share, and transport. Even viewing one file over a network can be difficult at times. When integrating systems, it's important to consider how each individual system affects the overall performance and capacity of the entire health system. You need to know the technology footprint of each system to effectively interconnect and integrate it into a platform that can oversee how it performs, such as AIOps.

As you can see, there are many building blocks to each and every piece we add and subtract to the entire convergence puzzle; however, this is the easy part. Once all systems are interconnected, and converged and can be used together, aspects of AI are intertwined into every one of these distinct yet now interconnected systems. Here are some of the pros and cons of AI when used across a fully integrated set of systems:

- Each and every one of these separate systems normally has AI and ML functionality built into it. For example, an EMR needs to be used by a doctor who may be busy doing something with a patient. If the doctor is too busy to stop and jot down notes in the EMR, they might use speech recognition software to take notes and add them into the system. The EMR and the speech recorder each have AI functionality, but leveraging their convergence can produce more advanced machine learning functionality. For example, while conducting a basic physical exam, a doctor might use speech recognition software to note that bloodwork should be done, and the EMR might make suggestions based on the patient's history or compiled data from similar patients.

- Another example may be the use of a patient portal. The patient portal is used when a patient (customer) needs to book an appointment, look at their most recent lab results, find a specialist, review their medication list, request new medications, and so on. The services provided are incredibly dense. Many times, a bill needs to be paid, or an inquiry needs to be made where assistance is needed. A telehealth appointment may be made and initiated directly from the patient portal. Every aspect of providing care and the way patients see data and connect to the system needs to be considered and safely provided. Every portion of this platform is provided through not only interconnection, but also integration of the systems and convergence of services that provide each function. AIOps can ensure that everything is event and fault monitored and is also set to automate functions, self-heal, promote automatic responses, and initiate proactive help as needed.

Note that Figure 9.2 shows the typical patient portal layout that, if designed correctly, can safely provide a patient the ability to access their latest charts and patient history, make appointments, and pay bills through integration and convergence.

TIP   Once all systems are connected and converged, you can start to leverage the benefits that tools such as AIOps platforms and service management service desks can provide. Self-help systems (such as catalogs of requestable services) can be offered from within the toolsets. This allows customers to request tools and services and even to ask for something that isn't currently provided.

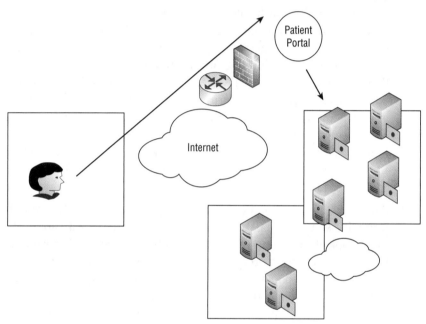

Figure 9.2: The use of interconnected systems

Convergence of AI, HIT, and HIE

Once you have interconnected and integrated your systems and have them all under the AIOps umbrella, you can start to dig deeper into the convergence of AI with healthcare IT (HIT). The Internet of Things (IoT) becomes the focus of current technology trends, making the automation of actions needed by the patient important. As we learned with the COVID-19 pandemic, automation of tasks, remote monitoring, remote assistance, and reacting (and sometimes acting proactively) to issues in a timely manner are all essential.

The focus on healthcare and service delivery as a whole is important and so is reliable and nonproblematic system performance. When we look at automating services, we look at how we can bring automation and services together under one central control, which is AIOps. The area where AI and AIOps overlap is fault and event management.

Healthcare information exchange (HIE) is the interconnection of all healthcare delivery systems for the purpose of exchanging information between them. This helps to service population health (pop health), increase revenue, and build better clinical outcomes by sharing critical information between disparate systems that need to work together to provide better healthcare.

Figure 9.3 shows an example of how an HIE can share information between different electronic health records (EHRs), EMRs, and other services to interconnect for the purpose of increasing services for all involved. Health information exchange can help to provide interconnection between different organizations worldwide. HIE is not a new concept. However, with the convergence of systems, it brings the ability to fuse artificial intelligence (AI) and machine learning (ML) into the HIE for new capabilities.

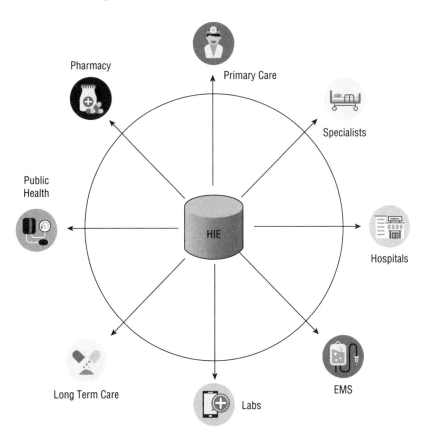

Figure 9.3: The convergence and use of HIE

The basic idea of HIE is to allow for clinicians, patients, providers, and recipients of care to be able to go anywhere in (and in some cases out of) the network and have access to critical data and services. The most important thing to consider when using HIE is that all major healthcare systems look to leverage this and, in some cases, even become HIE providers for other systems. That said, AIOps is one of the perfect tools that you can use to overlap all of the interconnected, integrated, and converged systems so that if at any time there is a break in the chain, it can be handled with AI technology for automated self-healing, keeping patients and clinicians able to use the data that they rely on.

> **TIP**   Business intelligence (BI) platforms are in high demand in healthcare systems. The ability to leverage data across systems provides for big data access to data that can be analyzed and reviewed for insights. Being able to protect the stability of this pipeline is where AIOps provides the best value.

IoT and AI

Once we start down the path of the Internet of Things (IoT), we learn that everything that is connected to a network becomes a thing that can be managed. (This is true regardless of whether the connection is wired or wireless.) Further, your AIOps platform can manage all assets across the IoT spectrum. Two of the fastest-growing converged technology groups are IoT and AI. Neither is new, but they both have matured and in the past couple of years have begun to merge or converge.

The most common form of AI and IoT convergence is the current use of smart home technologies. Smart home technologies often use voice-activated devices that can make decisions based on trends. A simple example of this would be setting up Google Home with AI technologies. In this case, Google would know when you need to set up a shopping list and alert you, when certain devices (such as security cameras) may be picking up anomalies, or when you should be dimming the lights before bed on a Monday evening.

All of this seems commonplace today in most technologically integrated homes, but what about in the hospital room setting? In the healthcare field, many tools, systems, technologies, and devices are used in the same way. Now, patients can get the same level of smart home innovation directly from their hospital bed where they spend their time receiving care.

But the convergence of AI and IoT extends far beyond what the patient experiences in their hospital bed. AIOps can track inventories of stethoscopes, surgical masks, and other medical equipment and notify medical professionals when supplies dip below a certain threshold. Emergency medical technicians (EMTs) can coordinate their efforts with their own companies, hospitals, and information databases. Implantable cardioverter-defibrillators, home insulin meters, and daily blood pressure can be synchronized between a patient's daily personal life and their doctors and specialists. Information from clinical research and cutting-edge trials from far-off labs can be fed directly into the AIOps system. Thanks to the convergence of AI and IoT technologies, all of this information can be integrated in your system. See Figure 9.4.

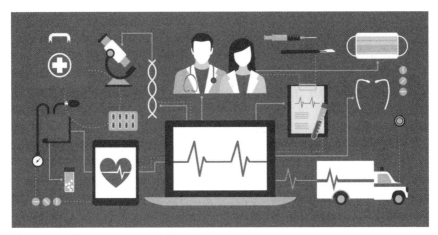

Figure 9.4: The complexity of IoT in healthcare

It is remarkable how many "'things" can be considered interconnected and converged and thus require management by a tool such as AIOps. This is where value can be discussed, that is, how to bring more ROI from your investment in AIOps. Most tools such as ServiceNow, for example, come with the ability to support and manage the IoT and can snap into the bigger architecture of AIOps for machine learning opportunities and advanced automation. Before we explain the "how," it's important to understand the "why." There are many challenges to managing assets that are distributed across the enterprise.

TIP   The use of a service management tool such as ServiceNow is important in providing a central nervous system to your technology. For example,

> if you want to be able to connect the IoT to your AIOps platform, you need to have all devices connected to the CMDB as CIs and have valid assets in your asset management program. Without this baseline configuration being put in place, all of the things you look to manage may be elusive and complicated to track.

As we discovered with COVID-19, another challenge is that we need to recognize emerging needs, deploy more IoT technology, and manage it correctly.

- There is a need to deliver healthcare to patients at home. Whether due to an aging populace, the need to remain socially distanced, or other reasons, there is a new need to create the ability to deliver healthcare directly into the home. There are many scenarios where this would be relevant to monitoring and managing vitals, tracking medications, and/or ensuring that there is a protective barrier that minimizes exposure of healthcare aides visiting the patients.

- There is a new need to keep the bedside protected and first responders safe. The ability to create wearables, wireless scanners, temperature readers, and other IoT devices, and the ability to manage them, collect and aggregate data to a central point, and use that data is important to future use cases and provider safety.

- Innovation is at its highest peak when looking at how the use of the IoT is managed by AIOps and how using AI and ML technology can be leveraged in a way to produce better outcomes. In Figure 9.5 we can see the use of HIT leveraging the IoT in a NICU for a clinician to care for a baby safely with multiple monitors and sensors fusing the technology of bedside devices to the central network for monitoring and management. This way, if any device (thing) has an issue, it can be proactively or reactively handled via fault management alerts and alarms.

The Internet of Things (IoT) also leverages the use of the Internet where any device anywhere can be used in the network. This can make management difficult but not impossible. You can also assume that if your AIOps platform is cloud-hosted, it too must be reachable by IoTs.

The cloud is important in this scenario because you may have your AIOps management systems hosted in the cloud. The ability of the IoT technology to connect remotely to these systems is incredibly important for their sustained functionality and security. When we are able to connect the devices in use to a management system that can employ AI to make decisions based on usage, you create opportunities for automation and self-healing technology. For example, if a device fails, it can be immediately seen on the AIOps dashboard as a triaged incident. An alert can be sent out to those who are monitoring and managing the system. Diagnostic checks can be done by the system prior to the ticket being picked up by an agent and tests run to bring the device back online. Either the device is brought back online or the agent is alerted to the problem and can have someone respond to the device to replace or fix it if needed.

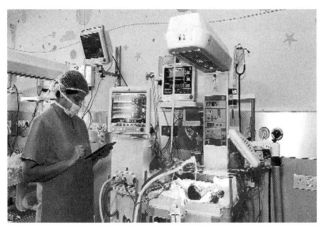

Figure 9.5: Using IoT in the NICU

Once everything is connected and manageable, this is where the true artificial intelligence (AI) solutions begin to develop. Voice technology systems allow for someone at the bedside (perhaps the patient or the clinician) to speak and the device to be able to respond to the requests. For example, if someone needs help, speaking to the device would alert those who need to know what help was needed.

When this technology is mapped to other devices in the room like monitors and health-related wearables, the entire picture of how AI can be leveraged starts to take shape. If a patient is a diabetic and their blood sugar levels are dropping, the IoT can provide the most value to the patient. Figure 9.6 shows a typical blood sugar monitor and an insulin pump that are connected as part of the IoT.

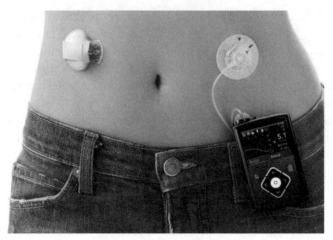

Figure 9.6: Use of an insulin pump and meter

Although this is something that the patient needs in the hospital or bedside, that doesn't change when they are discharged and go home. As an outpatient, the need to manage their health continues. Here is the entire scenario and how IoT, AI, and AIOps can provide the overarching technology that delivers the best care possible:

1. A patient is admitted to the hospital due to a minor accident where they may have broken a bone and need to have it set. The patient has underlying problems with T1D and needs to have their blood sugar monitored and insulin added to make corrections.

2. When brought in for handling by specialists who need to set the bone and handle that issue, vitals and other specific concerns such as monitoring blood sugar levels need to be handled at the bedside. These are done via the IoT, devices, wearables, and other technology all connected to systems monitored and managed by AIOps systems.

3. During the patient's stay, there is a power problem on the floor of the hospital where the patient is staying and the router sends an alert to the AIOps platform that there is a disconnection alert. A ticket is created for the issue, and the router is failed over to a secondary gateway allowing for the continuation of services without any impact to the patient or technology.

4. While in bed, the patient doesn't feel well and believes that they may have low sugar and need to have their sugar levels checked. The patient speaks into the Google Home device in the room and

asks for help, saying that they may have low sugar. The device can access the network that remained up and is able to securely review the patient's medical records over an encrypted channel. An alert is also sent to the nurse station to get someone to attend.

5. The wearable is able to inject insulin to make the correction and all monitoring data is collected and added to the health record but also given to the nurse to assist with monitoring and ensuring that the patient is stable.

6. All data is collected, the identifying information is depersonalized, and informatics are run via big data collection to see how we can better treat those who stay with T1D in the hospitals based on the most recent 100 cases over a period of 90 days.

Although this may seem like a lot, all of it could span the entire technology investment you have made to create a viable healthcare technology setting that allows clinicians to do their job with the help of technology but also gives patients the ability to get more out of their experience during their stay while in the system. Figure 9.7 shows that as the patient is in the hospital, it's the IoT framework that allows them to have the flexibility that they need to get the best level of care, but also shows how clinicians can leverage these benefits. It also shows how all of these systems connect back to datacenters to provide system access, services, security, data collection points, and many other services to allow IoT to function correctly and safely. It also shows how AIOps is used to help provide an oversight via fault and event management to keep systems operational. At all points AI is used to make decisions, self-heal, and provide more innovation via big data, informatics, and so on.

This example shows how AI and ML can interoperate with all other devices and how a voice-activated request turned into a workflow that required the action of correcting blood sugar to take place. There are many aspects of how AI and ML worked in this instance. For one, the IoT wearable was able to see that a low sugar level was occurring and that it needed to send an alarm. Normally, if at home, the alarm would be audible, and it would send a signal to a separate monitoring device or smart phone. The AI function algorithm would be: "IF low blood sugar and IF recorded at this level, THEN submit insulin from insulin in this amount." Using a Boolean workflow algorithm that simplifies actions from machine learning algorithms, it is easy to determine through trending data on a timeline (what blood sugar looked like that day, week, and month) and from analyzing this data that the patient is likely to record lows before lunch. This first-person, first-agent algorithm is intended to create an action through analysis. The algorithm is simple in terms of what the reaction (or proactive tasks) would be. Over time this data can be correlated with other data, such as a digital food log, to identify whether the patient's blood sugar goes low due to an influx of fiber in the morning with breakfast, and the patient is likely either not taking enough or taking too much insulin, and this should be changed moving forward.

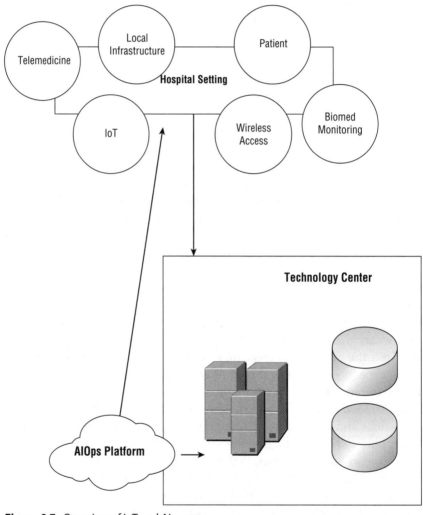

Figure 9.7: Overview of IoT and AI usage

This is the new age of bedside (and home-based) technology monitoring for healthcare service delivery but also for proactive care. Health systems have moved to new payment models where re-entry into a hospital can impact the bottom line. Caring for the patient at home especially after discharge is important to the viability of healthcare systems. Also, with threats such as a pandemic and the spreading of germs, more telemedicine delivery and use of the IoT are becoming increasingly prevalent every day. The tool used to make sure that all data is stored, safe, secure, reliable, and resilient and can be acted upon in any threat, issue, or outage is AIOps. This platform allows you to monitor all devices, systems, and functions smartly; it allows the clinicians to continue to provide care; it allows the patients the ability to have and keep access to needed services; and it gives peace of mind to all involved that AI can help to automate actions to keep systems up and running in times of crisis or issues.

IoT Management

IoT management is becoming more prevalent in all industries, not just healthcare. Industrial devices have been and continue to be retrofitted with intelligence that allows them to connect to networks and become part of the IoT. Because of this, more and more AIOps platforms become part of that equation to help manage the many assets that are in the workplace. With Splunk, there is the ability to manage, monitor, and review diagnostics of things that are connected and have faults associated to them. Monitoring and diagnostics are two of the most important management tools that can be provided when there is a fault in the system.

Data collection and analysis is what can be done with the information provided by the IoT devices. For example, reverting to the healthcare scenario, when we had a bedside medical device experience an issue, a fault can be sent to the system for collection and handling. Data collection and analysis provides operational visibility, proactive monitoring, operational control, and the reactive ticketing and assignment of problems that can be handled quickly and effectively. With healthcare, that can be a life or death situation in some instances.

A tool like Splunk can also provide the IoT with a predictive analytics ability based on collected data that is reviewed and shows trends on specific items. For example, if we have a fault show up for a specific device, it can be emphasized to those reviewing the data that you may have an issue with that device. These failures can be seen in fault detection, which can use audibles or other failure criteria that can be reviewed and corrected as necessary. IoT intelligence and automation with ServiceNow (SN) is similar to Splunk.

IoT devices report to systems and servers that manage them directly. See Figure 9.8. From there you can see how a tool like Splunk or SN can sit on the AIOps platform, collect data, and be able to alert on any failures to the devices themselves or the servers they connect to. The use of intelligent automation allows any break in this chain to be detected and handled. For example, if a wearable fails and reports to the server it is connected to that it is not responsive, the AIOps system can cut a ticket for the lost asset. There has been an interesting development where all software assets have been registered and can function with management software, but now with the IoT and the ability to develop new software for application programming interfaces (APIs), just about anything that can be networked (or made to be networked) can be connected and made part of the asset's management system and thus manageable via AIOps.

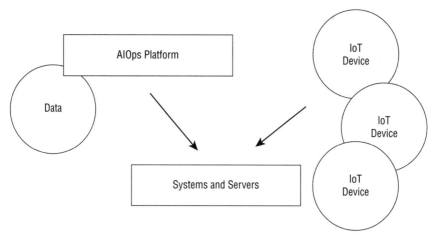

Figure 9.8: IoT management with AIOps

With ServiceNow, an IoT device can be integrated into Flow Designer, as shown in Figure 9.9. When using ServiceNow's IntegrationHub and Flow Designer, you can create the connections to the IoT hardware-based devices that need to be integrated into the system for fault management.

You can use the AI of IntegrationHub to incorporate, process, and use the data of the IoT devices that otherwise would normally be difficult to add. Using APIs and other integration tools and full automation of services together with autoremediation through engine-based actions can be established.

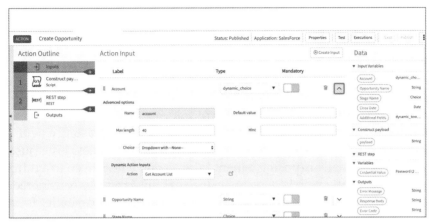

Figure 9.9: ServiceNow Flow Designer

Tools such as AIOps bring some of the only options to the table for creating a framework where workflows can be developed for the IoT and allowing for AI to become part of the process. Because the traditional smart home and personal mobile phone management of such devices is the basis for the beginning of how the new patient room will look, we can take a step back and look at the thousands of devices deployed and new ones every day that need to be ingested, managed, monitored, and automated via AIOps. True ML can take place and self-healing through learning from stored and analyzed data can become more of a reality.

REFERENCE   The IoT, although not a new technology, is growing every day. More devices are becoming network aware and need to be managed. AI is most effective when all of these devices are overseen by converged and integrated systems under the management of an AIOps system. Once all these parts are in place, true ROI can be established, but more importantly, the door to the world of innovation swings wide open for new possibilities.

AIOps Management and Security

As more devices are connected and used, this brings the world to an interesting place where security becomes problematic if it cannot be maintained. A major outage of Garmin wearable devices that wreaked havoc across the health field happened recently. There are two main reasons why I bring this up and why it is incredibly important to consider when deploying the IoT, AI, AIOps, or any piece of technology for that matter. When applying security to technology, there is an old saying that you cannot entirely secure something that you intend to use as a service. When you use something as a service, it opens it up to those who are invited in to access it. Yes, you can secure it, monitor it, and maintain security as much as possible, but providing the public with a service is always risky at some level. In healthcare, things are considered very risky when patient information is at stake. One of the main reasons why the cloud is scrutinized so carefully by those in the medical field is because you are potentially exposing patient information when given to a third party. Although much is done to ensure that this is always considered, handled, and constantly reanalyzed, there is always a possibility for a threat to become a reality.

When Garmin was impacted, the wearables still functioned, but they were not able to register with the servers that maintained them. This posed an interesting problem because, although the hardware devices themselves were not immediately impacted, people's ability to check their health stats, which was a critical service, was affected. Imagine if a similar scenario happened with a digital pacemaker looking to keep a heart pumping correctly or an insulin pump that administered insulin when needed. There are literally hundreds of similar "what if" scenarios where services could be hacked, hijacked, and ruined over ransomware.

The Garmin attack was simple. There was a way for hackers to get in and take control over the infrastructure that hosted the services for Garmin. The ransomware program encrypted everything that it infected and spread itself until Garmin was forced to suspend services until it could restore or rebuild its infrastructure. In Figure 9.10, it is clear that, using this example, the IoT can be rendered useless unless there is a way to protect and manage it as well as constantly monitor it regardless of AI involvement. AIOps is used to help provide fault, event, and security management and preventative actions via an automated workflow.

Note that Figure 9.10 shows the disconnection between the IoT device and the main server hosting cloud causing the inability to use the device correctly. The device itself is not broken, but its usefulness is now limited. This is the exact scenario we want to avoid when dealing with health delivery services that can cause harm to a patient.

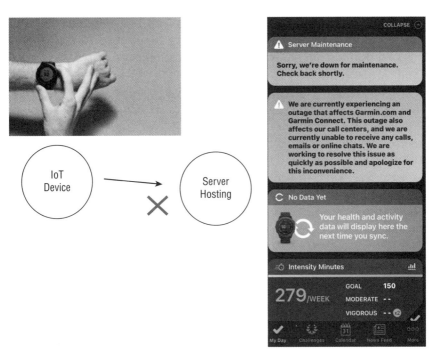

Figure 9.10: IoT and server failure

WARNING   Remember this example. When all of your systems are encrypted and someone is holding them for ransom, do you know what the most concerning things about this issue of exposure are? Obviously, the most concerning thing is the impact on your patients, including health risks and potentially even death. In addition, you suffer irreversible brand impact, embarrassment, and even legal action when you fail to secure people's private information. Loss of faith can lead to loss of customers. In healthcare, this can be extremely devastating and difficult to recover from.

There are things that you can do to ensure that your IoT infrastructure is secure with AIOps. One is to ensure that all devices are accounted for. The next step is to make sure that all infrastructure that is hosting services is also accounted for. Next, making sure that all of the devices are up-to-date and monitored for security threats is a priority.

While the IoT is an extremely helpful set of devices that allows us to do more with technology, it does increase our exposure to risk. Some of the other failures of this technology have also been exposed in the news and created brand and reputation damage. Baby monitor software with flaws in the software opened up spying opportunities. Digital locks on doors from smart homes that were recently upgraded with a software update allowed hackers to open them remotely. There are many stories of the IoT having problems, and although manageable, they were still problems nonetheless. With healthcare, the software must be closely watched, scanned, risk assessed, and monitored (AIOps) to ensure complete safety of the assets.

Figure 9.11 shows the sheer volume of devices, attack points, vectors, use case scenarios, and considerations. Remember, all of these devices can also move with the patient from location to location. Each device offers a point of access for an attack or threat. Risk must be considered at every point in the chain, and like any chain, it's only as strong as its weakest link. To remain secure, consider the following when you deploy IoT, AIOps, and other HIT technology into your infrastructure, environment, or home settings to practice healthcare:

- **Conduct a risk assessment.** Before rolling any of this technology out, you need to make sure that you have considered the threats. Do not become a Garmin. Make sure that you have assessed that letting all of this device functionality, inclusion of assets, and access into your network is safe and where your weak points are or may be.

- **Conduct ongoing assessments.** Penetration tests, vulnerability assessments, and other types of review of security posture can help to identify not only current but new threats. Many of these devices and their systems are considered safe, but then you have to update them. Patching, upgrading, or updating systems usually opens the door to a new threat, so constant assessment and tests need to be done to validate that ongoing security is functioning at a high level.

- **Standardize as much as possible.** It may be difficult to stick with one vendor or product brand, but when it comes to security, being able to hold the vendor accountable to produce patches or fixes for bugs and other security problems becomes problematic when there is someone else to lay blame on. For example, you may have an application that runs on a Windows server, and Microsoft may be called in to help validate where the break in the chain is.

- **Conduct a security project and harden your systems.** Make sure that you have allowed the appropriate access and nothing more. If you have overly loose security, it's going to allow something to wander in and create problems. Lowering your footprint, turning off services you don't use or need, and implementing other ways to harden are highly recommended.

- **Segment your IoT devices on to their own network.** If you have a way to create a segment for your IoT devices that need to pass through a monitoring firewall, use a VPN, and also be monitored by event and fault management via AIOps, you will be ahead of the game on extensive breaches that you cannot isolate the point of entry from.

- **Use management software to manage your IoT devices.** This is where a management tool and AIOps come into play. If you have AIOps as a platform and are able to incorporate your IoT devices into it, you can manage and monitor it as well as apply workflow automation that can also include security actions that can be taken if breached.

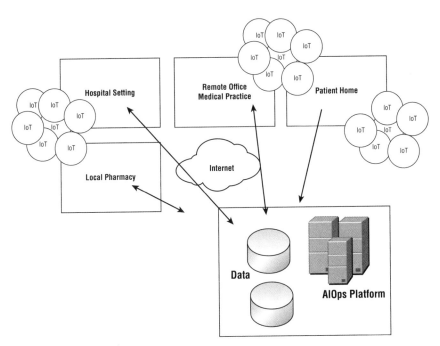

Figure 9.11: IoT attack vectors

WARNING   Security should never be an afterthought. Security should be planned from the beginning and implemented every step of the way when deploying any technology system into your enterprise.

There's another reason security is critical to the IoT and the future of secure AIOps. There are two major points of risk that we have highlighted throughout the book and primarily in this chapter, which are IoT and AI. When dealing with the IoT, you are potentially opening up a device to be hacked and taken over. With AI (and AIOps systems), you have the devices making decisions based on trends, workflow automation, dynamic proactive and reactive actions, machine learning, and other factors. When you put IoT and AI together, you have a pretty concerning situation if something is compromised. Now, let's take that "something" and identify what that might entail in the real world.

The healthcare setting needs to inspire trust in clinicians' decisions about patients' health. Data has to be reviewed, and decisions about administering care need to be made. The clinical staff has to trust that the data they use is reliable. Biomedical technology is one of the most interesting technologies in use today where the sensors used while administering care are recording data and feeding other systems that provide care, monitoring, and administering of medicine to the patient. When these systems are compromised or the wrong system data is fed into the system, both the trust in the ability for the clinician to make a good decision and the trust the clinician has in using the biomedical technology are at risk.

Figure 9.12 shows the connection of sensors that supply the clinician with information. For example, a cardiology patient with a pacemaker comes in for a checkup due to an issue they are experiencing, and an interface gets the required data from the device. An EKG also uses a set of sensors applied to gain valuable information for the clinical staff to make decisions. There are sensors that are outside the body, but there are also ones like the pacemaker that are implantable. Connected medical devices that are used to provide patient care can be at risk if the proper security is not used.

There also needs to be an analysis of the data before AI can be used as well. We do not want to use machine learning (ML) if the system is going to make the wrong decision and put the patient at risk. Patient safety is the number-one priority in all health systems. This why the healthcare industry has been slow to adopt healthcare IoT, AI, and ML. These technologies all converge and provide data for a great purpose, but we need to make sure that there are no mistakes. There have been crisis situations before, and devices have been compromised in the past. However, we have learned a lot from those experiences. We are now better prepared for the integration and convergence of all systems under a safe and secure AIOps system for overall fault, event, and monitoring management.

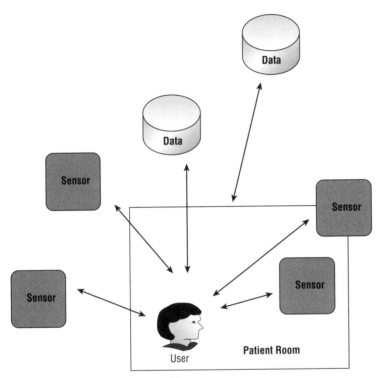

Figure 9.12: IoT sensors and healthcare

Summary

This chapter discussed the use of artificial intelligence, machine learning, and healthcare operations in an IT setting that leverages not only AIOps but other technologies and solutions as well to bring more benefits to the healthcare system. We have explored topics that relate to certain new technologies such as IoT and the ways in which AIOps can provide management and oversight to the growing number of devices and assets. Make no mistake, the Internet of Things is here to stay and will only grow exponentially. With this growth, we need to apply a monitoring and management system that does it safely.

Using AIOps extensively will help us integrate and converge systems holistically. AIOps platforms can become the center of everything and help you manage all of your disparate technologies from one place. AIOps also help you to bring in and connect one of the largest growing technologies in the healthcare information technology space, which is the Internet of Things. IoT, AI, ML, and AIOps are increasingly significant in delivering better healthcare by bringing together the integration and convergence of these and other technologies.

In the future, we will continue to see more healthcare technology evolve. It will be further integrated into existing systems, and convergence will allow us more benefits than we have seen in the past. With AI, we can create intelligence in every part of the enterprise that AI-enabled devices exist. As we have seen with HIE, IoT, and other high-level initiatives to create more ROI for health providers, the core of the return of that investment is ease of use as well as the reduction of issues and outages. With machine learning technology, we can provide an example of how things can be used together to create long-lasting benefits. With AIOps, we can supply the oversight to it all in a way that gives us the advantage of creating a safety net of management, monitoring, security, and action on demand. The future of healthcare is bright, and in the center of it all is a great AIOps system that helps to enable it all. The convergence of healthcare AI technology will help us bridge the gaps and make future innovation a reality for the leaders, technologists, clinicians, and patients who embrace it.

Sample AIOps Use Cases and Examples

Artificial intelligence for IT operations (AIOps) is an overarching system architecture that ties all of your interconnected systems together and uses machine learning (ML) to apply artificial intelligence to help make operational decisions in your environment. Machine learning uses and processes large amounts of data (big data) from your infrastructure, services, applications, appliances, devices, components, systems, tools, data, and other sources of information such as configuration management databases (CMDBs) and information technology asset management (ITAM) systems to give a holistic picture of your entire technology environment. You use that information to create automated functions and workflows and to make educated and strategic decisions.

The use cases provided help you take what you know about AIOps and plug it into a scenario that may be your own workplace or that of a future client. Regardless of which situation you find yourself in, you will discover that most implementation scenarios are unique and have multiple requirements that need to be understood and met. You will want to plan your AIOps system wisely and create a project charter and project plan to help guide you through your AIOps system deployment so that nothing is missed and you budget for it correctly. Your resources, time, and budget need to be understood and managed accurately since most of these deployments are costly not only in terms of money but also in time and effort.

AIOps platforms are used to help identify trends. When anomalies occur, AIOps platforms highlight them as a potential differentiating behavior from the normal processing of your systems. Performance data usually shows specific trends. For example, a bandwidth can hit a higher threshold when everyone is busy during work hours and be less used during the weekend when backups are the only thing that may be running on certain links. In this appendix, we will look at AIOps implementation and make sure that it's running correctly using the primary goals of all AIOps platforms as a marker for success.

- Is the AIOps system able to use machine learning to make decisions that are new and not based on old thresholds set in the past?

- Can the collected data start to expose new anomalies that have not been identified in the past?

- Can we find the root cause of an issue based on the AIOps platform's findings?

- Was the AIOps platform's AI functionality enabled, and did an automated workflow take place based on a decision made by the tool?

- Was an incident ticket created for the event? How was it handled?

- Did a postmortem review of the event show any deficiencies or lessons learned beyond those identified by the people who manage the system?

As we will see, the use case scenario plays out in a way where we can ask each question and identify whether our AIOps platform performed well. If it did not, we can determine what needs to be done to rectify any flaws or gaps for the future.

Scenario 1: Failing Application

"Failing application" sounds very generic, does it not? It is meant to sound generic because that is how our scenario starts. The help desk has received calls from frustrated and irate physicians who have tried to look at X-rays but were unable to because they received an error on the system. The first thing that comes to mind as a technology leader in a healthcare system is, why did the investment in AIOps not help find, identify, and perhaps fix the issue in real time? This is not an uncommon question to ask when a significant investment is made in technology that does not do what it is intended to. Similar questions can arise if you did not set expectations correctly, and leadership erroneously believes the system should have functioned beyond its currently intended scope.

Let's break down this scenario to uncover what the issue was here, why the problem was not identified, and if it was, why it caused an outage to a critical system and impacted the delivery of health services from clinicians across an entire hospital floor.

Identification

The first step in our journey of answering these questions is to identify what happened. This is probably documented in the system itself, especially if you are using a service desk system like ServiceNow. For example, if you had a failing application, a few things likely happened when the failure occurred. First, a disruption in service appeared, and then those who relied on that service escalated the problem to the IT department. Traditional methods for doing this include help desk calls, emails, chats, messages, and complaints to supervisors.

After the initial triage of the issue takes place, you can further refine your approach to include any and all information known about the issue, such as the location, the event, the expectations, and the general reason for the call itself. Odds are good that as you work on this issue, additional complaints will continue to come in. For each one, an incident ticket is created, and this information is prioritized based on the severity of the issue. If the application is servicing multiple sites and locations, you may get an influx of calls raising the call volume metric and the queue in the help desk to a high level. This will immediately clue you in on the fact that you have a priority 1 incident. If that is the case, then you will need to have the ticket routed to the correct parties to resolve it. The incident management team (which is the traditional service management team in the ITIL framework) will manage the incident to completion. Once this takes place, teams can converge on a call bridge and begin to resolve the issues and notify the client and management about what the problem is and when it will be resolved. Once this entire process is completed, the ticket will move to problem management where a root-cause analysis (RCA) can be done to identify what the true cause of the issue had been.

Postmortem

Once the problem is identified and corrective and preventative actions are put in place to fix the issue, the final step should be a discussion on what happened and how to prevent it from happening again in the future. This discussion should also consider the reasons why certain systems fail and the possibility of a more systemic problem existing. Being proactive about issues occurring again by trying to prevent them should be the goal of a good postmortem. Whether AIOps was used or whether it should be recommended to be used may be good topics to address. Questions that could be asked include the following:

- Was there an event and fault management system in place, and did it miss identifying the issue with the failed application? In this case, the answer quite simply is that the application itself failed (it had a bug added from a new service update from the vendor) and had nothing to do with the underlying infrastructure. AIOps was used, but it would not have been able to identify the application failure from an update to the code. AIOps should have seen it if the update was logged in the CMDB. What AIOps did see is that there was a performance problem, and it opened a series of tickets on the database, but it wasn't the root cause of the problem.

- Is the AIOps system able to use machine learning to make decisions that are new and not based on old thresholds set in the past? In this scenario, if the problem had been with the database, it may have been identifiable via thresholds that the AIOps platform had been monitoring. Exceeding thresholds could have created a warning event that someone could have investigated. In this instance, the code upgrade immediately caused a problem with the application. Therefore, the alerts from the AIOps platform came later, after the initial failure.

- Can the collected data start to expose new anomalies that have not been identified in the past? Yes. In this case, since the underlying infrastructure was already being monitored, it would have likely picked up the problems proactively and may have been able to map new anomalies that need to be considered in the future to keep the entire mapped system stable.

- Can we find the root cause of an issue based on the AIOps platform's findings? Yes, we were able to find that there was a problem. However, the root cause was not identifiable due to it being a problem with the application itself. Since the application was not covered by the AIOps system, that would be something to consider for future updates via the RCA and preventative (or corrective) assigned actions.

- Was the AIOps platform's AI functionality enabled, and did an automated workflow take place based on a decision made by the tool? In this case, there was no automatic self-healing process or workflow that could have taken place. What was found in the review of the postmortem is that the application resided on only one host and was not redundant or resilient. Business continuity planning (BCP) should be considered for this application's future upgrade plans. If a failover system had been available and implemented, AIOps might have been able to identify a problem, activate the failover system, and resolve the issue.

- Was an incident ticket created for the event? How was it handled? An incident ticket was created for this event. However, it was routed over from the help desk as an escalated priority. There were no high-priority tickets generated from alarms from the underlying infrastructure.

- Did this postmortem review of the event show any deficiencies or lessons learned beyond those identified by the people who manage the system? Yes, there are lessons learned that must be considered. For one, the application itself is not resilient. Also, as shown in Figure A.1, it's been reviewed that the application has further been identified as a cloud-hosted system that does not fall into the realm of our AIOps coverage. Although the AIOps system could have identified problems with multiple calls on the firewall, which caused it to degrade in performance from the retransmission of packets, it did so as a secondary event to the original failure cause. The root cause was an upgrade done by the vendor to the hosted application, which caused the impact. Further review shows that the hosted application change did not go through the company's change control process. Therefore, the only methods of identifying the issue were through the failure causing a high spike on the help desk and secondarily the AIOps system flagging anomalies at the firewall. Since the AIOps system could not learn why the issue was taking place, it could only alert via email and open incident tickets on the firewall itself. Both conditions helped technicians quickly find the source of the issue to be the application itself.

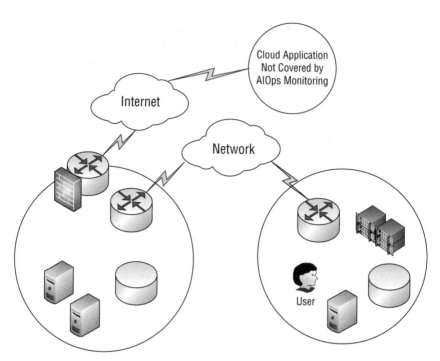

Figure A.1: Review of failure map

This use case scenario shows a common situation and demonstrates how a large investment in an AIOps system would not have been able to do much in this situation. Many times, companies host systems with vendors that cause disruptions. What is good about having an AIOps system in this situation is that you can quickly identify and rule out your own enterprise being the source of the problem. As the firewall indicated issues in degraded performance, there was an obvious reason why, and it could have been identified through fault and event management review. That said, the true AI benefit could not be realized in this instance. Over time, if this issue happens again, machine learning will start to track this anomaly, and there may be a future workflow that could create a self-healing situation, such as a secondary vendor in an alternate location that the system can reroute too if a performance hit takes place or if the service itself is disrupted and no longer available.

Scenario 2: No Access to EMR

In this next use case scenario, I take you through an event that causes a series of clinicians to have no access to their EMR. To further define the scenario, the ICU team at one of the health system's hospitals cannot access the electronic health records for their patients on the floor. The time of incident is at approximately 1 a.m., on Sunday morning, and several things have taken place. The clinicians seem to have noticed the outage, and at around 1:15 a.m., the access to their EMR had been restored. During the 15-minute outage, clinicians took notes on paper and then had to backfill them into the system at a later time. Downtime procedures did not have to take place due to the quick resolution of the problem. Because there was a break in service, the unit's head nurse made a call to the help desk to open a priority 1 ticket. The agent had informed her that the desk was aware of the problem. However, the ticket would be created so that she could call back and reference it if she needed. The on-call teams were mobilized due to alerts generated from the enterprise systems (Citrix Server load balancer) that there was a failed node. However, resiliency within the system was able to restore service quickly. The on-call engineer ensured that the system was stable and set the ticket to be monitored for 24 hours. The RCA was conducted, and it showed that although there was a break in service, it appeared at first glance that all systems operated as they should.

Let's break down this scenario to uncover what the issue was here, why the problem was quickly resolved, and how the service was brought back to the hospital's ICU department in a timely manner.

Identification

In this use case scenario, we need to look at what happened so that we can identify if AIOps played a role in helping solve this issue. Although the problem was resolved quickly (in less than 15 minutes), there was a break in service. It was also good that the clinical staff (head nurse) had called and the ticket was already opened and in work. It was also helpful that a ticket was created as a master ticket and each call that came in could be added as a child ticket to the main ticket for further review and identification. In this situation, it appears that AIOps was in fact used to help solve this issue through an automated workflow. Further review of the system shows that the fault was picked up in one of the network routers that connected to a remote site data center where the Citrix server farm was hosted internally to the health system and managed by the company's IT staff. The Citrix server farm was also serviced by a series of load balancers that could distribute requests for the applications it hosted. This particular server farm hosted the applications for the ICU group of the hospital that was impacted. It was later found that other hospitals were also impacted but the application had only been used in that 15-minute outage window by one particular hospital's ICU.

Postmortem

The investigation revealed the following relevant facts. All systems across the entire enterprise were covered by APIs and agents via the AIOps system. When the router failure occurred, the redundancy in the systems allowed for business continuity to take place and a failover condition to reroute the traffic. Although the system itself was resilient, the AIOps platform expedited the failover by seeing the anomaly, reporting it, and setting the automatic workflow in place to cut a priority 1 master ticket, correlate any child tickets, alert the on-call failover to the secondary node as soon as a failure condition was identified, and, in this case, remap the clients to the application via the Citrix ICA client program. The load balancer was not the source of the issue.

Further review of this issue required more questions for the RCA to conclude how the AIOps platform could have done this quicker and if the 15 minutes could be shortened in a failure state.

- Is the AIOps system able to use machine learning to make decisions that are new and not based on old thresholds set in the past? Yes. In this instance, the routers that connect the clinical staff to the hosted applications were redundant and had multiple connections to the data center where the application is hosted. When the outage took place, the router link dropped, and the router immediately reported the downed interface to the AIOps platform as a priority 1 outage. Once this happened, the automated workflow from trends gathered over multiple months showed that this has happened often and the exact same outage took place before. The system knew to immediately force a failover to the secondary node that would have rerouted the traffic to the application and reconnect the Citrix ICA client to bring the ICU applications back online.

- Can the collected data start to expose new anomalies that have not been identified in the past? In this situation, yes, that is precisely what it did. This was a recurring problem that has caused the same issue before. The administrator of the AIOps system should be reviewing metrics to see what can be done to permanently fix the issue. The problem management team should have an RCA that maps to older RCAs with open corrective and preventative actions that still need to be resolved. If the issue is with the network service provider, it needs to be addressed with them.

- Can we find the root cause of an issue based on the AIOps platform's findings? We were able to find the root cause from the AIOps platform. The router lost network signal from the service provider, and the router sent that information to the AIOps platform for action.

- Was the AIOps platform's AI functionality enabled, and did an automated workflow take place based on a decision made by the tool? Yes, it did. It took the appropriate actions to solve the problem.

- Was an incident ticket created for the event? How was it handled? An incident ticket was created for this event, had the correct priority set, and was handled quickly.

- Did a postmortem review of the event show any deficiencies or lessons learned beyond those identified by the people who manage the system? Yes, many of them. For some leaders this could have been seen as a victory. An investment was made in an expensive AIOps system, and it worked as advertised. The one thing that could not be understood without digging deeper into the problem was, why was there a 15-minute outage if everything was redundant, resilient, and covered by an enterprise AI-based management platform? The answer is that the AIOps platform needs to be tuned, and some of the information may not have been machine learned. For example, the actual incident that took place was an application outage caused by a router link problem. The root cause of the issue was that the service provider had a problem on their internal systems which caused a disruption to the service. The 15 minutes of extra downtime was caused by a failure to recalculate the routes because of a flapping condition that was overlooked and not part of the workflow for the AIOps platform's actions. For example, as shown in Figure A.2, there are two routers on the same service provider. A better solution to create resiliency would be to have two separate network service providers. What the RCA uncovered was that the service provider actually had an internal routing problem that caused a flapping condition inside their network that disrupted both links. Until it could be resolved, there was a disruption of approximately 15 minutes. AIOps could not have identified the problem because it's part of a vendor network and the secondary router appeared to be up, running, and available to handle the routing functions. As we have learned, this is another source of an issue that we may not have been able to find within our own AIOps framework.

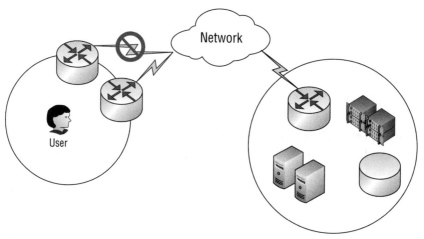

Figure A.2: Network resiliency

The two specific use cases that I used as examples in this appendix could help you immensely as you make progress on your AIOps platform deployment, management, and monitoring journey in your environment. AI is not the answer to all of your questions, it's only an answer to some of them. There are always more questions and always more answers. Machine learning is mathematical and works on logic. There will be things that come up to test that logic, for example, vendors that fall outside your ability to monitor. These can cause challenges to your ability to respond to issues. I chose these two scenarios because in a perfect world AIOps will do an outstanding job making your life easier, but we do not live in a perfect world. This should help show you that you should never take your eye off the road. You can let the car self-drive, but you need to pay attention to where it is taking you. AI and ML are really great technologies, and when used correctly, they provide massive benefits, but be aware of what they do not do as well. This way, you will also be ready for what is next.

> **TIP**   It is important to be able to talk about issues in this format. Leadership will want to know what the problems are and how you resolve them, how the systems resolve them, and what must be done next. To be able to articulate issues in this format will help you build confidence in the system as well as in those who run and maintain it.

Summary

As we have learned throughout this book, artificial intelligence for IT operations is used as an overarching system architecture that ties all of your interconnected systems together and uses machine learning to create artificial intelligence to help make operational decisions in your environment. Because there are many examples in which it can be used, these use case scenarios should help you with the language you may need from time to time to help you articulate what happened and what the system is capable and not capable of doing.

Index